# PSYCHIATRY AND HEALTH

# PSYCHIATRY AND HEALTH

## A Comprehensive Integration

**Jules H. Masserman, M.D.**

*Professor Emeritus of Psychiatry
and Neurology
Northwestern University
Chicago, Illinois*

*Honorary Life President,
World Association for Social Psychiatry*

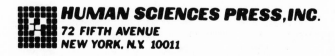 **HUMAN SCIENCES PRESS,INC.**
**72 FIFTH AVENUE**
**NEW YORK, N.Y. 10011**

Printed in the United States of America
987654321

**Library of Congress Cataloging in Publication Data**

Masserman, Jules
  Psychiatry and health.

  Includes indexes.
  1. Psychiatry. 2. Mental illness. I. Title.
  [DNLM: 1. Health. 2. Mental Disorders. 3. Psychiatry.
WM 100 M415pb]
RC 454.M2935   1986      616.89      85–14361
ISBN 0–89885–256–0

*To Christine*
*My Ultimate Tribute*

# CONTENTS

*Foreword*                                                          *11*

*Acknowledgements*                                                   13

1. **Definitions and Integrations**                                  **15**

2. **Historical Perspectives**                                       **20**
   Classical Roots                                                   21
   Ur I: To Restore Self-Confidence and Physical
        Well-Being                                                   22
   Ur II: To Recultivate Social Relationships                        23
   Ur III: Surcease in Comforting Faiths                             25
   Hebraic, Christian, and Islamic Contributions                     26
   Intellectual Emancipations                                        27
   Later Developments of Psychiatric Therapies                       28
   American Developments                                             29

3. **The Clinical Examination**                                      **34**
   The Past History                                                  38
   The Mental Status                                                 42
   Psychiatric Significance of the Physical
        Examination                                                  44
   Supplementary Psychologic Testing                                 44
   Ancillary Techniques in Psychiatric Diagnosis                     45
   Psychiatric Formulation                                           45

4. **Classification versus Diagnosis in Psychiatry**                 **47**

5.  **Preview of the Dynamics of Therapy**               **56**
    Comparative Experimental                              56
    Essential Modalities of Clinical Therapies            58
    The Essential Dynamics of Therapy                     59

6.  **Introduction to Therapy**                          **63**
    Responsibility                                        64
    Preconceptions                                        66
    Resistances                                           67
    Frequency, Duration, and Cost of Therapy              68
    Semantics                                             69
    Couples, Family, and Group Sessions                   71
    Termination of Therapy                                72

7.  **Hypnosis**                                         **73**
    Susceptibility                                        73
    Technique of Induction                                74
    Evaluation                                            75

8.  **Psychoanalyses**                                   **77**
    Theories and Therapies in Modern Dynamic
        Terms                                             77
    Psychoanalytic Concepts                               78
    Techniques of Psychoanalytic Therapy                  88
    Modified Analytic Techniques                          89
    Deviationist Schools                                  90

9.  **Diverse Dyadic Therapies**                         **95**

10. **Behavior Therapies**                              **104**
    Techniques of Therapy                                105
    Recent Critiques                                     107

11. **Group and Metapsychologic Therapies**             **109**
    Group Analytic and Behavioral Techniques             109
    Metapsychologic and Religious Modalities             116

12. **Pharmacologic and Somatic Therapies** **119**
    Alcoholism 119
    Psychopharmacology 124

13. **Psychiatric Disorders in Physically Ill**
    **Patients** **133**
    Psychiatric Manifestations of Physical Illness 133
    The Brain 134
    Endocrine Disorders 136
    Reactions to Physical Illness 137
    Treatment 139

14. **Therapy at Various Ages** **143**
    Review of Principles 143
    Infancy 145
    Childhood Neuroses 148
    Puberty 148
    Adolescence 149
    Sexual and Marital Problems 151
    Therapy in the Middle Years 153
    The Climacterium 154
    Problems of Aging 156

15. **Clinical Illustrations** **161**
    Case  1: The Penurious Man 162
    Case  2: Somatization Disorder; Amaurosis 163
    Case  3: Obsessive-Compulsive Disorder;
            Familial and Religious 163
    Case  4: Atypical Somatoform Disorder with
            Marital Therapy 164
    Case  5: Counterphobic Reaction 165
    Case  6: Anxiety-Phobic Disorder with Homicidal
            Panic 166
    Case  7: Sociopathic Personality Disorder;
            Progress to Criminality 168
    Case  8: Conversion Neurosis; Military
            Implications 169

Case  9: Atypical Impulse Control Disorder with
          Alcoholic Delirium and Dysthymia        172
Case 10: Midlife Adjustment Disorder; Rapport,
          Reorientation and Resocialization        174
Case 11: Psychophysiologic and Affective Disorders
          with Schizophrenic Channelization        176
Case 12: Schizophrenia with Symbolic Dereism      179
Case 13: Hypomania Following a Prolonged
          Depression                               182
Case 14: Psychogenic Pain Disorder                185
Case 15: Geriatric Personality Disorder;
          Therapeutic Rehabilitation               186
Case 16: Family Therapy; Forensic Aspects          186

16.  Review and Integration                        **190**
*Appendix 1: DSM III Classifications*               193
*Appendix 2: Glossary*                              205
*References*                                        241
*Index of Names*                                    245
*Index of Subjects*                                 249

# FOREWORD

This book summarizes over 40 years of study, research, and teaching in psychiatry, including its origins in anthropology, history, sociology, and esthetics as well as in comparative and clinical psychology, medicine, and psychoanalysis. In presenting a synthesis of these disciplines I have avoided recondite terminology, esoteric theories, and pejorative controversies in favor of comprehensive dynamic principles and integrative approaches to diagnosis and therapy. The volume is therefore intended for everyone, from students to specialists in the humanistic sciences, who shares its ideals of brevity, clarity, and cogency.

I shall ever be deeply grateful to the geniuses in my field, among them Adolf Meyer in psychobiology and Franz Alexander in psychoanalysis, who enlightened and inspired me. I am similarly indebted to the many colleagues and friends credited in the text who collaborated in my research, helped integrate my thoughts and practices, encouraged my previous writings, and prompted this summary volume. May it fulfill their expectations and those of its prospective readers.

# ACKNOWLEDGEMENTS

To have furnished no specific references to the hundreds of books and articles cited would have made the text appear unsupported and dogmatic; to have listed all the original sources would have increased the size of the volume beyond reasonable limitations. The option reached was to refer readers interested in pursuing selected topics to publications by the author or others in which the subject was sufficiently developed for most purposes and referenced for fuller investigation as desired.

Thanks are due to the American Medical Association, The American Psychiatric Association, Grune & Stratton, Inc., Intercontinental Medical Books, Jason Aronson, Inc., Thieme-Stratton, Inc., Charles C. Thomas, Inc., and W. B. Saunders Co. for permission to adapt limited segments of my previous publications to the purposes of these volumes. Herewith also my special appreciation to John J. Schwab, M.D. and Clifford C. Kuhn, M.D. for the data reviewed in chapter 13. Additional technical terms are defined in the Glossary.

*Chapter 1*

# DEFINITIONS AND INTEGRATIONS

Psychiatric terms have often been regarded as so vague or ambiguous as to impair clarity of thought and application. However, there is an inherent philologic and semantic wisdom in many key concepts, exemplified in the two selected for the title of this volume. For example:

*Psyche*[1] is Greek for *mind*. But if "mind" is regarded as a *process* rather than as a substance, three dynamic determinants of human behavior emerge. Thus:

We *mind*, i.e. perceive and adapt to our environments through the media of our somatic (bodily) systems.

We *re-mind* ourselves of past *ex-periences* (i.e., those that have significantly "pierced through") to put current ones in context, and

We *mind*, in the sense of obey the accumulated requirements of our sociocultural milieu.

*Iatros* is Greek for physician: in psychiatry, a person trained and dedicated to restore *patiens* (Gk., sufferers) to "mental" as well as physical optimum functioning.

*Health* stems from the Anglo-Saxon roots *hâl* or *hōl*, again with three significant derivatives in modern English:

From *hâl* comes *hâle*, connoting physical well-being, strength, skill, and endurance. Failing these, *healing*, in the sense of spontaneous recovery or medical intervention, must take place.

From *hâl* also spring *hail*, *hello*, *heil* in German; (*salud* "health to you!" in Spanish), all having the import, "Salutations, my friend, I wish you well!" Humans, as social beings, must ever cultivate interdependence; ergo, a corresponding objective of therapy is to guide the patient in developing or restoring essential alliances.

Third, from the root *hōl* have come *wholesome*, denoting culturally integrated and approved, and *holy*, denoting an adherence to acceptable faiths—two other objectives of therapy.

The single term *health*, then, comprises the fulfillment of the three universal and ultimate (Ur) needs of mankind. Briefly stated,[2] they are:

*Ur I, Somatic*, for the vitality, operational skills,[3] and longevity necessary to control the physical environment,

*Ur II, Interpersonal*, for social hegemony and security, and

*Ur III, Existential*, for reassuring beliefs in an ambient philosophic or theopoetic system.[3]

Correspondingly heuristic also are the following terms:

*Personality* stems from the mask through which a Greek actor spoke (*per-sona*) while playing a prescribed role. So also in modern usage, personality may refer either (a) to the public facade beneath which a person conceals his true identity or (b) to a cultural stereotype.

For example, the comment that someone has "a good business personality" may mean in our current culture that he or she is calculating, preemptive, smooth, competitive, opportunistic, and perhaps even dishonest but shrewdly within the law. Conversely, an unambitious, modest, reserved, socially overconscientious, and sensitive individual would have "personality difficulties" in some of our commercial or political enterprises, but in this context it might be contended that it is the social system, not the individual, that needs revision.

*Disease* refers to a state in which a person feels discomfited, alienated or troubled (i.e. dis-eased), as to his somatic functions (Ur I), interpersonal relationships (Ur II), or cherished beliefs (Ur III). *Illness* is more directly derived from evil-ness.

*Diagnosis and Prognosis* (L. *dia*, thorough, *pro*, fore-, *gnosis* knowledge) therefore transcend the mere naming (nosology) of a dis-order through re-cognizing its physical, social, and metapsychological causes and manifestations and its probable outcome.

A significant corollary of this parameter is that there is hardly any deviation called a *neurosis*, a *sociopathy*, or a *psychosis* in our culture that would in some other time or place be considered not only normal, i.e., within its norms, (mores or morals) but actually admirable.[4] For example, on the physical plane, a dermatologic affliction called *pinto* is so common among some Amazonian Indians that anyone not having it is socially ostracized. Behaviorally, gentle passivity sometimes to the extreme of masochistic fatalism is advocated by the Zuni, some Hindu sects, and the Society of Friends; paranoid belligerence and easily aroused violence are wisdom to the Dobuans; epileptic seizures or catatonic stupors are evidence of divine possession in many religious cults, and throughout the world, what one person regards as ignorance and superstition, is another's holy faith and sacred ritual. This makes available a great variety of climates, occupations, and sociocultural environments to suit a wide range of individual preferences. To take a whimsical example, a troubled and troublesome American bigamist could, Mormon Utah being no longer apt, be counselled to move to Abu Dhabi, Kuwait, or Kenya, become a Muslim, marry four wives and, provided he also conformed to other local customs, live quite "normally" ever after.

*Therapy.* This ultimate term (Gk., *therapeien*, service) further clarifies a threefold task. First, if patients are handicapped by somatic illnesses or neurologically by sensory, mnemonic, associative, and motor impairments, every medical or surgical means to restore these somatic functions must be employed.[5] Second, if patients have also developed socially inappropriate conduct, they must be helped to reexamine and reevaluate their aberrant past and current patterns of action as being neither as necessary nor as advantageous as they had, consciously or not, assumed them to be. Concurrently they can be guided toward new interpersonal and cultural adaptations that, through further experience, they will choose to maintain as ultimately more practicable and profitable.

As may be inferred from the above, three corresponding modalities of therapy have emerged: organic-individual, socioadaptational, and metapsychologic, with many "schools" in each category. However, each school or subcult has advocated a separate theoretic system in a new terminology[6] (or, worse, has attributed differing meanings to the same terms) and has attempted to prescribe supposedly unique methods of therapy on the presumption that new modalities were more scientific, efficient, or fundamental than those based on older concepts. The multiple modes of therapy so derived will be discussed in chapters 5 to 15.

## NOTES

1.  In Greek mythology, Psyche was the name of a lovely maiden visited nightly by a mysterious lover who lavished gifts and affection on the sole condition that she never learn his identity. However, overcome by a spirit of Freudian research one dark night, she lit a candle and discovered that he was the god Eros. For this she was condemned by Olympus as an eternal admonition to mere humans—especially indiscreet mistresses—to keep their illicit erotism covert. In Greek poetry Psyche (as mind, spirit, or soul) was also represented as an iridescent, delicate butterfly, reminiscent of the philosopher Lao Tse, who dreamed he was a butterfly, and ever after wondered if he was a butterfly dreaming he was a man.

2. Hence *Homo habilis*, the (mis-) user of tools, but not necessarily *Homo sapiens*, man the wise.

3. Michelangelo's wondrous painting in the Sistine Chapel can well represent Adam giving life to God.

4. J.H. Masserman, *The Range of Normal in Human Behavior*, 1976.

5. A whimsical clinical fantasy relevant to systems theory can epitomize the linkages among somatic, interpersonal, social, and potentially global vectors of human behavior: a pathologic dysfunction in the islets of Langerhans of the pancreas (*organic* level) causes diabetes on the generalized *somatic* level, resulting in impotence on the *symptomatic* level that may eventuate in *marital* dissatisfactions, uxorial unfaithfulness, and *interpersonal* jealousies with possible *social, legal* and, even homicidal complications. Further, when powerful persons were involved (e.g., Menelaus of Sparta, Phillip of Macedon, Henry VIII of England), devastating conflicts on the *international* level resulted that could conceivably have been prevented, had insulin and calmer counselling been available on the *therapeutic* level.

6. Rarely in accord with Occam's famous Razor: *Entia non sunt multiplicanda praeter necessitatem*, modernized by Garrett Hardin as the Principle of Parsimony.

*Chapter 2*

# HISTORICAL PERSPECTIVES

*Evolution may be re-viewed as a tentative account of how living organisms, by biodynamic interactions, strive to attain physical integrity, collaboration for species survival and, in the case of man (and possibly in some related species, e.g. dogs) comfort through superordinate faiths.*

After over three billion years of prevertebrate, vertebrate, and humanoid development, our species had attained the physical and psychological potentials we have today, plus a growing arsenal of tools with which to extend our skills. So too, men had assumed apportioned roles in group protection and hunting, women in food-gathering and child care, and together in other mutually serviceable endeavors. But since this still did not provide adequate security in an unpredictably dangerous world, they also developed wishful beliefs that they could further control their fate through symbolic fetishes, totems, and rituals.[1] As examples, they carved mammiferous amulets ("paleolithic Venuses") which apparently symbolized a deified wife or mother; so also, neolithic paintings in chapel-like caves (as in Altamira and Lascaux) apparently represented prayers intended to ensure the success of the forthcoming hunt. And as to concepts of immortality, Mousterian men were buried along with their weapons, wives, and utensils in expectation of a domestic life thereafter. In essence, then we had (although ever asymptotically) striven to attain the three ultimate and universal ("Ur") objectives previously outlined:

*Ur I for Survival and Control of the Physical Environment*. All of medicine is still a quest for strength, competence and longevity, and through other sciences we seek to extend our powers over the material milieu.

*Ur II for Human Alliances*. Insofar as this has been effective, we have expanded our allegiances from the family through the clan, tribe, and nation to the distant vista of world brotherhood; but insofar as this has failed, larger and larger tribes by more lethal means have tried to exterminate each other, and may yet succeed.

*Ur III Cosmic Control*. But even could we master our planet and pool all our capacities in a global society, would we still appear to be only an ant colony on an insignificant pebble mocked by a vast, impenetrable, and indifferent universe? Perish the thought: instead, we are the Chosen People of a God who devised all Creation for our special benefit; indeed, since He is our Omnipotent Parent, we can secure earthly comforts and eternal bliss thereafter by various techniques of appeal, bribery, or (as a last resort) obedience that once worked well in our childhood.

## CLASSICAL ROOTS

When the primitive pastoral and agrarian cultures had developed sufficiently to establish centers of learning in Babylon, Egypt, Crete, and later, throughout the Aegean, many Greek geniuses clearly anticipated our modern modes of thought.

Anaximander traced evolution from inorganic matter to animals and men. Pythagoras identified the brain as the organ of the mind, approximated the functions of the nerves, distinguished higher "cerebral" from inferior "emotional" behavior, and derived mathematics and esthetics (especially music) from a harmonious universe. Plato, quoting Socrates, conceived of ideal forms in nature, surmised the purpose of dreams, and proposed a social hegemony based on (his) philosophy. Aristotle utilized both inductive and deductive reasoning and Theophrastus, his successor at the Athenian Academy, wrote an anthology (Chapter 15) of classical personalities[2] as intuitively perceptive as Thucydides' analysis of the motives of historical figures. Xenophanes accepted man's needs for anthropomorphic deities, while Epicurus derided fears of imaginary gods and demons. Hippocrates, "father of medicine," taught his students at Cos to avoid cant and superstition in favor of clinical objectivity and to adhere to ethical and humanitarian principles of therapy.[3] Heraclitus, long before Hegel, perceived the dialectic antitheses-syntheses between the rational and irrational in human conduct and, long before Camus, between life and death. In their Asklepiad Sanatoria[4] (*sonatos* = health, named for the son of Apollo, god of medicine and music[5]) the techniques employed addressed all three Ur- needs as follows:

## GREEK THERAPY
### UR I: TO RESTORE SELF-CONFIDENCE AND PHYSICAL WELL-BEING

After the patient had left his contentious home and traveled to one of the Sanatoria in the pleasant environs of Cos, Memphis, or Knidos, he was met by no less a personage than the Head Priest or Priestess, who welcomed him and enhanced his expectation of recovery by conducting him past piles of discarded crutches and bronze plaques bearing testimonials from grateful ex-patients. Attention was then concentrated on nourishing and appetizing diets, relaxing baths and massages, and the confident administration of medicaments that, though regarded by modern standards as ineffective or possibly harmful, nevertheless pleased both physician and patient. As described by Pliny the Elder, Egyptian and Hellenic physicians also induced therapeutic convulsions by having an electric eel discharge its current through the patient's head, or by trephining the skull and lobotomizing the cortex to expel choleric or melancholic humors. True, Plato condemned the "ignorance and superstition inherent in many of these false remedies," but this alone indicated how widely practiced, then as now, variously partially effective or placebo therapies must have been.

## UR II: TO RECULTIVATE SOCIAL RELATIONSHIPS

Physicians of the School of Cos were also taught to elicit and correlate the patient's unique experiences with past and current illnesses (i.e. secure a psychiatric history) and then to provide wise and empathetic counsel as to healthier and happier modes of living (*v.* the Stoic schools). To practice these reorientations ("insights") the Asklepiad sanatoria utilized the following modalities of therapy:

Calisthenics and dancing for interpersonal coordination;

Music, for esthetic expression and feelings of conjoint rhythm and harmony (Chapter 13);

Dramatics, in which basic human relationships were sensed in the readings of classic poetry or in witnessing or acting the comedies of Euripides, Aeschylus, and Sophocles. Here the Greek myths of Psyche (Chapter 1), Narcissus, Electra, Oedipus, et al. conveyed deeper insights into the infinite interplay of human desires, fantasies, and foibles than do their current simplistic eponyms. For example, Narcissus was not "in primary love with himself" as implied in the Freudian term *Narcissism*; instead (on reflection), he grew so enamored of his idealized *image* that he forsook his friend Almeinas and his appropriately named mistress Echo and became as his Nemesis a flower child. Again, whether or not, as Eugene O'Neill would have it, mourning became Electra (cf. Ferenczi's "father-daughter complex") it became fatal to her mother Clytemnestra, to her mother's lover Aegisthos, to her brother Orestes, and to practically everyone else involved.

But far beyond these, perhaps the most inclusive and poignant of man's perennial vicissitudes are dramatized in Sophocles' trilogy on Oedipus—a succession of legends which, instead of epitomizing only a son's supposed desires for coitus with his mother countered by presumed fear of castration by his father's terrible swift sword, deals much more poignantly with nearly all human travail and triumph, through infantile survival of parental rejection, youthful seekings and fragile attainments, to futile adult quests and ultimate appeals to the gods for forgiveness and immortality:

Laius, King of Thebes, is warned by an oracle that his son by Queen Iocaste would slay him—as, indeed, all children will inevitably displace their elders. To avoid the direct onus of infanticide, Laius instead hobbles his child (as many parents vicariously now do) by pinning his ankles together (Oedipus: swollen feet) and, there being no bulrushes about (as in the legend of the Babylonian hero Engidu or the Hebraic Moses), leaves him in a basket on Mount Cathaeron. In this myth, Oedipus is rescued by the kindly shepherd Tiresias, who arranges to have the child adopted by Polybus, King of Corinth (as many of our own rejected children are rescued by baby-sitters, nursery school teachers, and other parent surrogates). But Oedipus is never certain that he is really the legitimate Prince of Corinth, does not accept assurances from King Polybus or Queen Merope (can anyone be *absolutely* certain of his paternity?) and is further perplexed when he learns at Delphi that he is destined "to kill his father and marry his mother." Trying to escape his fate (as who does not?) he vows never to see his putative parents Polybus or Merope again, and leaves Corinth to wander in search of what, in a current solecism, would be called his "true identity." At a crossroads outside Thebes, an old man disputes his right-of-way and is killed in the ensuing battle (as all elders who challenge our imperious youth will be disposed of in their turn). Then, to display his intellectual as well as physical supremacy, Oedipus also conquers a Sphinx whose "riddle" (the ancient nursery puzzle about man's successive quadri-, bi-, and tripedal locomotion) he easily solves, and thereby emancipates the Thebans from years of sphincteric terror. For reward he is given the throne of Thebes vacated by King Laius (whom Oedipus had *unknowingly* slain), and the privilege of marrying the widowed Iocaste.

But since nagging doubts remain (who does not have them?), Oedipus, after more years of restless questioning (the curse of Western man), learns from the now aged Tiresias the awful truth that he had indeed killed his father Laius and cohabited incestuously with his mother Iocaste—"awful" only because he fears that others regard it so. With appropriate histrionics, he blinds (not castrates) himself in expiation (and thereby secures the advantage of being a pathetic rather than a reprehensible figure), curses his unwanted sons Eteocles and Polynices, and preempts the lives of his daughters Antigone and Ismene (as countless aging parents have done) to serve his declining years. Finally, at the Grove of Colonus he justifies his behavior before Athena and Apollo, defies death, and himself becomes a demigod—thus acquiring the archangelic status we all believe our due.

There are, of course, many variations of these legends, not only in Greek, but in Hungarian, Roumanian, Finnish, and even Lapland folklore. In one classic version, Homer has Iocaste commit suicide, after which a more sensible Oedipus completes his reign in relative peace. But the stories are never naively monothetic to the Greek listener or patient; instead, they still illuminate our own childhood insecurities, our later seekings, temporary triumphs, and wishful resolutions.

## UR III: SURCEASE IN COMFORTING FAITHS

Finally, in accord with this third necessity, even the sophisticated Greeks demanded that Socrates pay the ultimate penalty for questioning man's trust in the existence of anthropomorphized and glorified celestial beings. In the temple attached to each Sanatorium and dedicated to Zeus, Apollo, or some other Olympian god, prayers were said, sacrifices were offered, and rituals were supervised by duly empowered priests to secure health, fortune, and eternity for compliant votaries. Among the intents and practices:

1. Conjoint experience of the "spiritual"—a concept as fundamental to existence as the neonate's first breath (L. *spiritus*, breath, soul). During life thereafter, he may become *inspired* to achieve both personal success and a social participation through an *esprit de corps*; failing both, he would become *dispirited* and *desperate* enough to seek physical, social, and metapsychologic help until he *ex-pires*, when his spirit leaves for parts wishfully imagined.

2. Temple hymns, sung and played in the simple, repetitive cadences of a lullaby, and often ending in a revitalizing or malleable "temple sleep," analogous to an hypnotic pseudo-trance (Chapter 8).

3. The "laying on of hands" and "anointing" to cure a malfunctioning bodily part—directly reminiscent of the soothing parental stroking of an injured child; still sought from masseurs, chiropractors or from tactual "sensitivity experiences."

4. The symbolic eating and drinking of the parent-god's body in the forms of mystically potentiating food and wine, as derived from the ancient worship of Melitta and Mithra.

Classical insights into human Ur-needs and therapies survived the fall of the Greek and Roman empires and, through Christian monasticism and Islamic scholarship, the Dark and Medieval ages into the Enlightenment.

### HEBRAIC, CHRISTIAN, AND ISLAMIC CONTRIBUTIONS

The ancient Hebrews (in the tradition of the Hindu Vishnu versus Siva, or the Taoist *Yang* versus *Yin*) conceived of an eternal struggle within man between *Yetzer ha'Tov*, the spirit of good, and *Yetzer ha'Rah*, the spirit of evil. To counter the latter, Yaweh had authorized Aaron and Moses to prescribe strict sanitary (Ur I), sexual and social (Ur II), and religious (Ur III) codes for the children of Israel that were to be followed on pain of disease or death. Nearly two millenia later St. Augustine, after he had tired of his youthful Manichaean diversions, likewise ordered inviolate rituals for physical health, Christian communion, and Ambrosian grace. Religious orthodoxy held sway both West and East, but was not unrelieved by humanism: Throughout Christendom (witness Fra Angelicus and Paracelsus) and Islam (witness Ibn' Sennah and Moses ben Maimon) next to churches or mosques princes, priests, and imams built hospices (hospitals) where sufferers were treated not only by the diets, baths, purges, medicaments, and surgery available at the time but also by human empathy[6] as well as by the essential comforts of religious faith. However it must also be recorded that inasmuch as some were judged not to deserve such compassion, in 1480 the

Dominican monks Sprenger and Kramer, with Papal sanction, published the *Malleus Maleficarum*,[7] a manual on how to detect evil-working witches who slew and ate children, spoiled crops, and otherwise harassed the devout. Despite the courageous protests of physicians such as Johannes Weier in Germany who wrote "my heart is tortured by such superstitions," and Duns Scotus in Britain, the diagnostic criteria and the recommendations for treatment (usually *auto da fé*) established by the Malleus resulted in millions of defenseless humans (including men of genius like Giordano Bruno or intrepid women such as Joan of Arc) being labelled servants of Satan and burned alive.

## INTELLECTUAL EMANCIPATIONS

Satan, unabashed, continued to send devastating plagues, while religious wars further decimated the population, so that only after Europe emerged from these nightmares could more thoughtfully anthropocentric philosophies emerge. Descartes wrote *"Cogito, ergo sum,"*[8] and Spinoza added "All the things I fear, and which fear me, had nothing good or bad in them save insofar as my mind is affected by them." Kant structured the world according to human "categorical imperatives," Schopenhauer more imperiously subjugated the universe to his Will and Idea; and Hegel dealt with such concepts both dialectically and synthetically. Nietzsche extolled the amoral Superman; and Goethe had the scientist Faust defy the Devil himself. Comte tried to reduce all human interactions to a mathematical science (Ur I), predicted the abolition of irrational politicoeconomic controls (Ur II) and ended by deifying and worshiping his dead wife Clochilde (Ur III). Spinzoa and later Kierkegaard submerged reason in favor of an intensity of experience that was at once an acknowledgment and a defiance of death—an existential stand that, with the added esthetic comforts, was also assumed variously by Santayana (who admired the "beauty of theology,") and, agnostically, by Sartre and Albert Camus. Kafka pleaded with man's unknown persecutors, while Thoreau sought escape in a bucolic Walden. More recently, Ernst Cassirer echoed Heisenberg's Principle of Uncertainty by asserting that man, whom he dubbed *animal symbolicus*, lives by cherished illusions and symbols rather than by "facts"—unless facts, as in *facit*, are what man makes of unknowable "reality."

## LATER DEVELOPMENTS OF PSYCHIATRIC THERAPIES

After the Reformation, a charismatic Cromwellian lieutenant named Valentine Greatrakes claimed that, without clerical or royal (King's touch) sanctions he could "purge the bodie of evil humores [by] skillfulle stroacking" alone. Thousands of people flocked to his "Greate Klinicke" to have this self-proclaimed healer "stroke" them, just as thousands today are certain they obtain relief from massage, chiropractic, or variations of Chinese acupuncture or moxibustion. A century and a quarter later, Anton Mesmer, a physician, based his system on the belief that when he touched his subjects, or merely made prescribed movements with his head or hands, he could deeply influence them to their (and his) benefit. Mesmer called this effect *animal magnetism*, analogous to both the "healing lodestones" on earth and the "astrologic attractions of stars and planets." Those of Mesmer's patients whom he could not treat by his personal magnetism would avidly surround a tub containing iron filings previously "magnetized" by Mesmer, fall into similar trances, have vivid and often erotic dreams, and awake claiming to feel vitalized, exhilarated, and "mutually emphathized"—much as occurs after "sensitivity sessions" today.[9]

Mesmer was eventually discredited and died in poverty, but his system, as noted, had resonated with so many Ur- longings that there sprang from it several of our current cults and practices, for instance:

The wearing of "magnetic belts," still sold by mail-order houses and believed by thousands of people to increase potency, cure diseases, and prevent debility.

Present-day hypnotism, in which practitioners with various degrees of wisdom or naivete perennially rediscover that many people like to depend upon and, within limits, obey a person who wields supposedly esoteric powers (Chapter 7).

The Christian Science Church, founded with fervent zeal and administrative genius by Mary Baker Eddy after Phineas

Quimby, an American mesmerist, "cured" her of various hysterical disorders. With consummate effectiveness, this Church invokes all of the Ur-faiths as follows:

*Ur I:* A simple, repetitiously assertive set of "health directives," all the more effective for their dogmatism. Christian Scientists assert "I stoutly affirm that I have no Dyspepsia, that I never had Dyspepsia, that I never will have Dyspepsia, . . . that there never has been any such thing, and that there never will be any such thing. Amen."

*Ur II:* An almost universal kinship through more than three thousand Churches of Christ Scientists, so that no believer need ever feel alone anywhere in the Western world.

*Ur III:* Church services which consist largely of readings from Mary Baker Eddy, endlessly reiterated, so that one feels familiar with all there is to know of a system of doctrinaire beliefs as propounded in its founder's book, *Science and Health with Key to the Scriptures.* This also reveals scientific as well as religious truths, among them, that a Christian Scientist is not confined to time or space, but can heal at any distance with semidivine power.

Predictably, a great many troubled, lonesome human beings join Christian Science churches or other organizations with similar faiths and rituals and thereby find precious relief and comfort. No one can deny the medical tragedies that can result from the misapplication of such doctrines and practices, but no one can gainsay the surcease afforded hundreds of thousands of people desperate for supposed physical relief, social contacts, and quiet faiths being offered. Nor, as therapists, can we neglect or deny anything that concerns and comforts humanity.

## AMERICAN DEVELOPMENTS

In colonial times, the "feeble-minded" or "insane" were pilloried, jailed, or expelled from their communities to wander the countryside, abused and abjured.[10]

However, after the reforms of Pinel and Esquirrol who

struck the chains off the inmates of the Bicêtre and Salpetrière Hospitals in Paris, followed by William Tuke in England, and Chiarugi in Italy, an Association of Medical Superintendents of American Institutions for the Insane was formed in 1844. Its early presidents administered hospitals in which Franz Joseph Gall's phrenology and C. Lombroso's "stigmata of degeneration" continued to be considered bases for diagnosis; but purgings and bleedings were moderated and supplemented by special diets, occupational therapies, and "moral suasion." Isaac Ray, President of the renamed American Medico-Psychologic Association from 1855 to 1859, pioneered forensic psychiatry and aided Dorothy Dix (1802-1887) and the Society of Friends in persuading legislators to transfer the mentally ill from almshouses or jails to properly built hospitals, where medical care, kindness, and "the inculcation of proper personal habits" were alleged to cure 80 to 90 percent of "the insane."[11] Various fads, such as homeopathy, injections of gold salts or cobra venom, and the removal of "focal infections," also emerged. The latter practice was exemplified at the Trenton State Hospital in New Jersey where Henry Cotton, its superintendent, claimed to cure psychoses by removing "cryptically diseased" teeth, tonsils, spleens, gallbladders, and even sections of intestines to cure hidden "auto-intoxications." As late as 1925, R.S. Carrol and H. Viner advocated the subarachnoid injection of horse serum to induce a reactive meningitis in psychotic patients, with claims of a two-thirds rate of improvement.

Fortunately, at about the turn of the century, American psychiatry had begun expanding its interests beyond hospital boundaries. In 1895, three years after his arrival from Switzerland, Adolf Meyer, on the basis of his research at the Kankakee State Hospital, criticized the prevailing concepts of mental illness as "unnecessarily fatalistic," and proposed more flexible constitutional-experiential percepts of etiology and therapy. Later, as head of the Phipps Psychiatric Clinics of Johns Hopkins (1912) and as President of the APA (1927-28), Meyer developed a comprehensive, diagnostic and therapeutic system called psychobiology. This organon substituted for stereotyped "mental diseases" the effects of deviated "life energies" ("ergasias") which were to be treated by suitable combinations of physiologic, interpersonal, and social-rehabilitative modes of therapy. Meyer also joined with Clifford Beers (a former mental patient who wrote *The Mind that Found Itself*) in organizing a national movement to which Meyer gave the name "Mental Hygiene" to signify the importance of proper familial, educational, occupational, and other salutary life experiences "productive of physical and mental health."

But another influence had become paramount. After the introduction of psychoanalysis to the U.S. (v. Chapter 9), and despite early schisms, Freud's theory of a pansexual or aggressive "Unconscious," and his presumed advocacy of intensive and prolonged "transference therapy" intrigued many clinicians. In 1911 the American Psychoanalytic Association was organized, and still operates under a rationale of orthodoxy. In 1955, the more broadly oriented and interdisciplinary American Academy of Psychoanalysis was founded by Janet Rioch, Sandor Rado, the author, and others to encourage more comprehensive research into the protean etiology and versatile therapies of various behavior disorders. Finally, the World Psychiatric Association, founded in 1964 by Pichot of France, A. Lewis of England, F. Braceland of the U.S., and others, and the International (now World) Association for Social Psychiatry, founded in 1968 by J. Bierer of England, V. Hudolin of Yugoslavia, G. Vassiliou of Greece, the author, and others, have organized worldwide scientific collaboration in their respective fields.

The resultant dialectic interplay of somatic, psychobiologic, analytic, and other modes of thought and practice in American psychiatry as advocated since 1878 by the American Psychiatric Association will be detailed in subsequent chapters.

But the theme of history remains: *Quo vadimus?*

## NOTES

1. W. Schmidt, *The Origin and Growth of Religion*, particularly pp. 283-291.

2. See Case 1, Chapter 15.

3. For a more detailed account of how Greek physicians anticipated in essence nearly every current psychiatric concept and

practice, see Masserman, *Practice of Dynamic Psychiatry*, Chapters 21–23.

4. However, with some trepidation, since Asklepios and his daughters Hygeia and Panacea were slain by Zeus for being too beneficent to mortal man.

5. For contrapuntal relations between the two, v. Masserman, *Say Id Isn't So—With Music*, 1964.

6. Wrote Angelicus in 1275 "Madness (and illness) cometh . . . of excess passions of the soul . . of great sorrow . . . of too much study . . . or of dread. (But) also by sweet accord, harmony and music, sick men and frantic come oft to their wit again and health of body."

7. The enthusiastic acclaim accorded the *Malleus Maleficarum* among the cognoscenti for nearly three centuries (and as recently reendorsed by the Rev. Montagu) may serve as an historical caution against concluding that "controlled field trials" of any "diagnostic manual" (Appendix 1) can establish its validity.

8. Lao Tze (Chapter 1) would have phrased it "I think, therefore I *think* I am."

9. In curious parallel with the current training of psychoanalysts, anyone could apply to a Mesmeric Institute for training to become "an Accredited Animal Magnetist" by being personally magnetized and magnetizing a number of subjects under officially "controlled" supervision. He was then certified as a Graduate Magnetizer and accepted into National and International Mesmeric Societies which published erudite Journals of Animal Magnetism, and could then treat people according to the Society rules. But if he tried newer and better methods, he was subject to a reconsideration of his "loyalty" and "professional qualifications." The Paris Academie de Médecine ruled that lay practitioners could magnetize only under medical supervision, but the edict was largely ignored by an initially enthusiastic public (J. Ellenberger, p.156). Mesmer, however, as was the case with Freud a century later, felt himself martyred by the medical establishment of the day and, despite adverse reports by a royal commission including

men as prominent as Benjamin Franklin, remained convinced that he had discovered a universal system of healing, as did many of his disciples. So he had, in the sense that he had again tapped basic human yearnings for physical repose, trusting human relationships, and mystic experiences that had been utilized in the temples of Mesopotamia and Egypt and in the Asklepiedae of classical times.

10.  In 1812 Dr. Benjamin Rush, whose likeness graces the Journal of the American Psychiatric Association, still held that, since "psychopathic behavior" was caused by disturbances of the cerebral circulation, it was to be treated by purging, blood-letting, "whipping when necessary," and "gyrators" or "tranquilizing chairs" to which patients were chained "to instill the curative fear of pain or death."

11.  Anticipating modern "rest cures," Weir-Mitchell (1830-1914) treated "neurasthenia" in well-to-do patients by regimes of prolonged confinement in darkened rooms, forced feeding, and the limitation of all "stressful activities or social contacts." After some days or weeks of this, many patients predictably decided that their life outside this institution had been more pleasant than they had previously thought.

*Chapter 3*

# THE CLINICAL EXAMINATION

As outlined in Chapter 1, patients appeal for aid when they feel that any one or all of their basic (Ur) needs are threatened, to wit:

> Their physical well-being is or is about to be impaired;
> Their familial, occupational, or other securities are endangered;
> Their previously cherished faiths no longer provide adequate comfort and serenity.

Correspondingly, the initial interview(s) should clarify the nature, intensity, and behavioral manifestations of these anxieties (diagnosis); their experiential origins and previous and recent exacerbations (personal history); the optimum modes for their favorable modification (therapy); and the relationships of the above to somatic, social, cultural, and therapeutic realities (prognostic vectors).

**The Setting.** The office should be comfortably furnished, quiet, and adequately soundproofed. Decorations may include reassuring diplomas and awards, photographs of easily recognized scientific or other public figures (e.g. Sigmund Freud, Albert Einstein, et al., jointly with the therapist if possible) and unostentatiously placed objects indicating the therapist's breadth of intellectual, cultural, esthetic, recreational (e.g., sailing, flying, exploring) or other interests, in one or more of which the patient may be a participant.

**Empathy.** As will be developed in Chapter 4, the therapist will recall that under stressful life situations he himself had reacted with excessive anxieties, obsessive suspicions and fears, minor depressions, and other deviations in thinking and mood with concomitant physiologic and behavioral manifestations. This will contribute to professional tact and understanding, sharpen the examiner's sensitivity to important clinical data, promote communication and confidence and, even in the first interview, lay the groundwork for effective therapy.

**Presenting Complaints.** Especially in the case of an acute anxiety state, the presenting symptoms may seem to indicate an immediate diagnosis of one of the syndromes described in Chapter 4. However, as detailed below, further inquiry will rarely, except for actuarial or other advantages, justify classifying the patient exclusively under any single DSM III rubric as listed in Appendix 1.

**The Current Illness.** In many instances the patient, even after medical referral, may still believe himself to be physically ill and initially resent any implications that his symptoms have other than a primarily organic causation. It is therefore often advisable to enhance the patient's cooperation by confirming that his or her physical and laboratory findings are normal. However, since a psychiatric disorder can never be diagnosed merely "by excluding organic disease" and the two are not mutually exclusive, *positive* evidence of personality, neurotic, and/or psychotic dysfunctions must be tactfully elicited. With the patient reassured that, happily, there is little or no indication of an organic illness (Chapter 13), he must be led to consider whether his symptoms could spring from other causes. Terms suitable to the individual (e.g., "overwork," "prolonged tension," "emotional strain," etc.) may be employed in these introductory explanations, while avoiding confusing or pejorative phrases such as "psychosomatic disorder," "nervous breakdown," or, worse, "mental disease." Most patients will then more readily accept the possibility of so-called "functional" or "emotional" factors in their illness.

**Modes of Communication.** The patient's choice of language may be idiosyncratic. Complaints of "headache," for example, may not indicate actual cephalalgia, but rather a sense of emptiness, oppression, or generalized discomforts vaguely referred to the "head." Other ambiguous terms favored by patients are "dizziness" (ranging from vertigo and slight faintness to syncope), "noises in the head" (tinnitus, obsessive sounds, or auditory hallucinations), "nervousness" (meaning anything from mild restlessness and hypersensitivity to uncontrolled furors), "sleeplessness" (troubled dreaming), "irritability," (temper outbreaks), "tensions," etc. However, challenging such evasions prematurely may elicit anxiety and resentment; so also, indications of secret drinking, sexual deviations, paranoid hostilities, etc. may be evident, but further explorations may be postponed until the patient's confidence has been secured.

**Circumstances that Exacerbate or Alleviate the Presenting Complaints.** The following data may be highly significant:

*Typical situations* in which anxiety, phobias, obsessions, and melancholic or paranoid reactions are evoked: e.g., when the patient is called upon to perform an unwanted task, when he is censured by some authority, or when he is otherwise rendered fearful, helpless, or hostile.

*Temporal correlations:* a wife's migraine headaches which appear only on weekends when she must contend with the continuous presence of her husband and children, or periodic impotence in a husband who unconsciously wishes to avoid impregnating his wife during what he presumes is her fertile cycle. The *nature* of the symptoms may be symbolic: gastric hypersecretion in immature, dependent patients, when they feel inadequately fed or cared for, or visual difficulties in potential voyeurs. However, in the absence of direct evidence, care must be taken not to make presumptions about "specific psychosomatic formulas."

**The circumstances under which symptoms are relieved** are similarly important: vacations, change of work or home, alterations in the family or social constellation, or hospitalizations. Particularly significant is the history that the patient had felt initially benefited by a wide variety of treatments administered by many therapists, but that in each case the "illness" returned as mutual enthusiasm flagged, after which the paient would seek another therapist with renewed complaints. This, of course, has a prognostic bearing on the patient's relationships and responses to any projected therapy.

Preliminary information may likewise be gathered about the deliberate or covert advantages the patient may derive from the illness. These may take the form not only of financial compensation and relief from responsibilities ("secondary or epinosic gain"), but may also satisfy security-seeking, regressive, covertly aggressive and other "primary" neurotic purposes.

**Precipitation of the Present Illness:** i.e., the special circumstances which, operating on a previously sensitized individual, served to precipitate the current symptoms. In the case of postcatastrophic neuroses the trauma may be fairly obvious; but more frequently, though the stresses involved were taken seriously by the patient, they are far less evident to an outside observer. In such instances they may consist of more subtle but equally disruptive threats such as a dreaded demotion or promotion, guilt (fear of punishment) related to another's misfortune, an impending but ambivalently regarded engagement or marriage, or various social or religious transgressions of special significance to the patient.

## THE PAST HISTORY

Since psychiatric disorders are exacerbations of previous personality patterns, it follows that these should be traced as fully as practicable from early familial influences through the vicissitudes of later life to the onset of the patient's current disabilities. However, many patients will be ignorant of, and unconsciously resist recognizing, any connection between their current difficulties and their past experiences.

**Transitions in Context.** If during his account of the present illness, the patient has vaguely or euphemistically described himself as "nervous," "emotional," "oversensitive," or "high-strung," he may be asked if these or other characteristics were familial traits, thus leading the patient to give significantly colored descriptions of his relationships with his parents, siblings, and relatives. Similarly, logical transitions may be made by inquiries whether current or other symptoms were present in childhood, and influenced by "excessive study in school," "overwork," or difficulties at various jobs or in military service. Information on particularly guarded topics such as sexuality may be more readily secured by an indirect approach: a complaint of dysmenorrhea may be a basis for asking the patient to describe her menarche; once the subject is broached, she may more easily be led to describe her sexual fantasies, predilections, traumata, etc. (See Sexual Development and Attitudes). Similarly, tracing a complaint of impotence or frigidity may reveal early erotic prohibitions, recourses to homosexuality, and related difficulties.

**"Irrelevancy."** The patient's surface diffuseness may reveal significant associative themes. For example, a patient may "wander" from an account of her marital unhappiness to a description of her idyllic childhood with her widowed father, or an aggressive competitive individual may dwell on his past mistreatment by those in authority (including, by implication, a warning to the examiner). As indicated, a completely undirected interview is rarely as informative as a skillfully guided one, but both techniques may be employed.

**Sources of the Past History.** In general, the patient himself will furnish the most significant data, but other sources may be utilized: interviews with family and friends, perusal of physicians', employers', or social service reports, school or military records. However, since all such sources have limitations and biases, each may require individual evaluation and comparison with others.

**Significance of the Data.** A psychiatric history endeavors to discern the *characteristic patterns of past and current behavior* that have diagnostic and prognostic value. The aim, therefore, is not merely to determine *what happened* in the patient's life, but *his concepts* as to his role in bringing the occurrences about, his subsequent responses to them, and how, consciously or not, these led to his present difficulties. Thus, there need be no overt striving for a precise "historical accuracy," since if the patient's accounts of past events are deliberately falsified, distorted, or replaced by symbolically wishfully imagined ("screen") memories, his verbal and nonverbal communications will be psychiatrically significant. In this sense, the proffered "history" is also an excellent index of the patient's "mental status," in that it furnishes valuable data as to his current motivations, fantasies, self-concepts, and interpersonal relationships.

With these qualifications, the information secured under the heading of personal history may be grouped within the following categories:

**Heredity.** Although genetics may play a role in the major psychoses, it is questionable whether there are significant hereditary factors in the neurotic behavior disorders. However, it is undeniable that the personality of every adult is greatly influenced by those with whom he comes into intimate contact, especially in childhood. Therefore, the patient's description of the personal characteristics of his grandparents, parents, siblings, or other relatives is often significant, particularly when special aspects of, or gross deviations in, their behavior (overindulgence, tyranny, unpredictability, neglect, hostility, sexual seduction) directly affected the patient's early environmental and formative experiences.

**Birth and Early Development.** Accurate data may be difficult or impossible to obtain, but the patient's or other informants' impressions about the following may be significant: prematurity; ease or difficulty in delivery (asphyxia, injuries); type of nursing and methods of weaning; delays in early habit acquisitions such as sitting, walking, word or sentence formations, and toilet training; early feeding difficulties; excessive crying; night terrors; tics; spasms; phobias; persistent thumb-sucking or enuresis; and encopresis. The above data are, of course, particularly relevant in the direct or ancillary examination of children and early adolescents, as supplemented by play, games, mutual story telling or other techniques.

**Sexual Development and Attitudes.** Tactful, objective inquiry into early sex preoccupations (autoerotisms, curiosities, fantasies, fears, inhibitions, displacements); later development; nature, pace, and intensity of homo- or heterosexual expressions; deviations in techniques or unusual attachments or aversions to sex partners. Previous and current marital adjustments including not only sexual compatibility, but also relative fidelity or promiscuity, use and justification of contraceptive methods, attitudes to in-laws and children (Chapter 15, Case 16), mutual interests and other interpersonal conflicts and satisfactions. In most instances, it will be found that these considerations *secondarily* determine sexual adjustments in marriage, rather than vice versa. How often or with whom the patient has sexual intercourse will be found to be less significant than for what purpose: self-reassurance, seduction, hostility, dominance, etc.

**Other habit developments.** concerning food, sleep, dress, hobbies, and, recreations. In later life, the survey should include habitual overindulgence in tobacco, caffeine drinks, alcohol, "tranquilizers," barbituates ("downers"), stimulants ("uppers"), "psychedelic" drugs ("pot," LSD, cocaine, mescaline, the especially toxic phencycledene "angel dust") or addictive narcotics.

**General Social Adjustments.** These include the type and constancies of friendships and group loyalties; submissiveness or leadership in joint activities; the nature and intensity of social, ethical, and religious sentiments with special reference to unusual rigidities or prejudices; and the circumstances leading to compatibility and belongingness, or, conversely, feelings of shyness, diffidence, embarrassment, resentment, alienation, and social failure.

**Occupational History.** Work sought or idealized; jobs secured and periods held; variability of effort and application; acceptance of duties and cooperation or competitiveness with fellow workers; idleness and failures; responses to supposed injustices or to promotions and successes; evaluation of employers, superiors, or employees. From this part of the anamnesis the examiner can determine the patient's prevailing cultural values or prejudices and the strains which accompany either social achievement, or failure and downward mobility.

**Military Service.** Dates; branch; reactions to training, discipline and combat; demotions and promotions; type, grade, and motivations at discharge; pensions sought and retained; current attitudes.

**Effects of Injuries and Illness.** An account of the patient's previous organic illnesses, including a description of significant reactions to them such as excessive invalidism, prolonged disability and dependency, or lack of cooperation under medical care and hospitalizations (Chapter 13). Accident-proneness and consequent litigation may alert the examiner to the possibility of malpractice suits.

**Transition to Present Illness.** Under this heading the past history may converge with the circumstances that, singly or in combination as outlined above, interacted with the patient's special sensitivities and vulnerabilities to precipitate his present illness, and to seek (or be referred for) psychiatric help. Not infrequently, however, a complete demarcation cannot really be made, and the "present illness" will be seen as merely a continuation, or, at most, an exacerbation of the patient's previous life patterns and aberrant tendencies.

## THE MENTAL STATUS

Since most patients will have only somatic, characterologic, or neurotic, rather than "psychotic" disturbances, crude tests of intellectual capacities, disorientations or hallucinatory experiences may be not only unnecessary but alienating. Actually, valid information as to most of the rubrics of the so-called "mental status" will already have been gathered during the course of the history and physical examination, as indicated by the following review.

**General Behavior.** The patient's appearance, gait, posture, demeanor, dress, personal hygiene, mannerisms, tics, characteristic activity, manifest idiosyncracies or compulsions, cooperation with office or clinic procedures, and general responses to the examiner and others.

**Intellectual Level.** This may be inferred from the quickness and relevance of the patient's perceptions, the versatility and specificity of his vocabulary, his capacities for both concrete and abstract thinking, the scope and accuracy of his general information, the richness of his imagery, his forms of wit and humor, and the general nature of his cultural attainments. In estimating basic intellectual capacities, however, allowances must be made for the previous presence or absence of social and educational opportunities.

**Mood and Emotional State.** The fixity or range of the patient's conations and affects: e.g., indifference, anxiety, depression, euphoria, hostility, etc., will have been in part verbally communicated by him during the interview. In addition, the examiner may have noted such physiologic and mimetic accompaniments as flushings, lachrymation, pupillary dilations, tremors, jaw-clenchings, muscular tensions, sudden startle reactions, and other visceral and motor expressions of various emotions. The stooped posture, slow movements, low retarded speech and dolorous facies of the melancholic are especially noticeable; in such patients, the possibility of self-destructive preoccupations may be better investigated gently and indirectly (e.g., "Are you sometimes so discouraged about your illness that you feel there is little use in going on?") than by challenging questions as to how (by drugs, gun, dramatic leaps) the patient plans to commit suicide. The examiner will also sense the touchy apprehensiveness of the anxiety neurotic, the bland "*la belle indifference*" of the so-called "conversion hysteric," the strained, restless pseudoeuphoria of the hypomanic, the demanding, self-pitying, nihilistic attitudes of the melancholic, or the dereistic, withdrawn affective distortions and deviant rapport of the schizoid or schizophrenic (Chapter 15 Cases 12, 13).

**Preoccupations and Special Symptoms.** When indicated, further inquiry may reveal persistent fantasies, significant dreams or nightmares, phobias, obsessive preoccupations, compulsions, hypochondriacal tendencies or fixations, diurnal or other variations in energy level or temperament, recurrent *déjà-vu* experiences, feelings of depersonalization, confusion or panic, and transient absences or prolonged fugue states (see glossary). Even more serious psychological deviations may incidentally be uncovered, for instance: hallucinations may be described in response to an inquiry about "very vivid day-dreams or imagination," whereas paranoid or other delusions may emerge clearly during the interview.

**Sensorium.** Memory, retention, associative and communicative capacities, orientation, etc., are not organically impaired in the neuroses. If, however, intellectual failures possibly due to cerebral trauma or disease are indicated by gross discrepancies in dates, places, and relationships in the history, the patient's sensorium may be further checked by indirect questions designed to reveal his awareness of identity, time, and locale, or his capacity to recall his past consistently. Only when specially indicated need the patient be requested to repeat forward or backward a series of from four to eight numbers, to subtract 7 serially from 100, to retell an anecdote, or to act adequately on a set of simple directions.

**Insight.** This is always a complex, relative, and variable aspect of the patient's past attitudes and current status. Clinically, insight may be estimated along the following dimensions: (a) the patient's own explanations of his illness, (b) his ideas as to prognosis and treatment, and (c) the sincerity of his desires for, and cooperation with, medical and psychiatric therapy. However, the ostensible acceptance of the examiner's favorite formulae may merely represent what Ehrenwald calls "doctrinal compliance" by the patient, and should not necessarily be regarded as indicative of true operational understanding.

### Psychiatric Significance of the Physical Examination

The patient's conduct during this procedure (Chapter 13), likewise contributes evidence as to his mental status: e.g., excessive shyness, modesty, or exhibitionism; extreme passivity; suspiciousness or hypersensitiveness with regard to abdominal, vaginal, or rectal examinations; or irrational fears of transillumination or retinoscopy. Incidental observations should include the adequacy of oral, ungual, and other personal hygiene, tattoo marks, drug rashes, evidences of minor scarrings from repeated syncope, or signs of hypodermic or intravenous use of narcotics.

### Supplementary Psychologic Testing

Whenever there are forensic, actuarial, or other special indications, the patient may be referred to a clinical psychologist for the following: (a) *Tests of intellectual functions*, such as the Wechsler Intelligence Scale or the Bender Gestalt, (b) *Tests of occupational preference or special abilities*, such as the Strong Vocational Guidance Scale, (c) *Personality tests* such as the "objective" Minnesota Multiphasic Personality Inventory (MMPI) and projective techniques such as the Rorschach and the Thematic Apperception Test.[2] The Masserman-Balken modification of the latter may be especially revealing.[3]

## ANCILLARY TECHNIQUES IN PSYCHIATRIC DIAGNOSIS

These include polygraphic recordings during questioning or history-taking ("lie detection"), hypnotic catharsis or regression, or the administration of drugs such as scopolamine ("truth serum") or intravenous sodium pentothal or sodium amytal (Chapter 12). With the possible exception of the latter, such procedures are rarely if ever necessary in psychiatric diagnosis, have no evidentiary validity, and carry definite physical and psychologic dangers; however, the physician should be acquainted with their general significance.[4]

## PSYCHIATRIC FORMULATION

This is designed to organize the information obtained into a clear and coherent summary which has explanatory value and relevance to diagnosis, prognosis, and treatment.

In essence the formulation should include:

A brief description of the patient and the succinct statement of the precipitating circumstances, nature, duration, and course of the present illness.

An evaluation of organic factors as revealed by the medical history and by the physical, neurological, laboratory, and other special examinations.

An analysis of constitutional and experiential vectors as indicated by the familial and personal history, and supplementary psychologic or other tests.

An interim diagnostic summary based on the above including: (a) the presence and *relative prominence* of various psychiatric syndromes (e.g., anxiety, physiologic dysfunctions, depression, schizoid tendencies, etc. (Chapter 4), (b) the relationship of these reactions to specific external stresses (environmental maladaptations), and (c) their roots in inner motivations, formative experiences, and derived character patterns (psychodynamics).

Indications for further medical or psychologic diagnostic procedures.

Preliminary plans for therapy, as recorded under the following rubrics:

Immediate symptomatic relief by medication, sedation, physiotherapy, or other medical or surgical procedures.

Environmental alterations such as a change of residence or work, or, if necessary, hospitalization for total care.

Projected nature and techniques of the therapeutic modalities to be employed (Chapters 5 to 15).

Methods of securing the cooperation of the patient's friends and family in his treatment or, when necessary, in his legally arranged custodial care. Later formulations should be elaborated and amended as other facts become available and new procedures followed.

The above would then constitute a comprehensive *diagnosis* (Greek: knowledge) of the patient rather than an ambiguous label (*DSM III*, Appendix 1) for the complexity of unique interactions among the therapist, the patient, and the relevant factors in their milieu.

## NOTES

1. *Note-Taking*: The examiner should be sufficiently familiar with the nature of the information he seeks to make it unnecessary to consult this or any other outline during the examination; to do so implies incompetence and impairs the ease, rapport, and effectiveness of the relationship. For the same reasons, it is best to avoid voluminous writing (or covert audio recording) during the interview, but brief notes may be taken of key observations for later elaboration.

2. Masserman & Schwab, 1976, pp. 75-104

3. Masserman & Balken, 1954

4. Masserman, J.H. *Practice of Dynamic Psychiatry*, Chapter 4.

Chapter 4

# CLASSIFICATION VERSUS DIAGNOSIS IN PSYCHIATRY

Carl von Linne (1707-1778) in his *Systema Naturae* attempted to classify all plants, animals and mankind by binomial terms of genus and species. August Comte (1798-1875) in his *Cours de Philosophie Positive*, held that such schemata were only way points between mysticism and science, and that no simple taxonomy could be heuristically relevant to the vast varieties of human characteristics. Instead, Comte propounded an organon he called "Psychologic Sociology" to encompass the almost infinite contingencies and vicissitudes of men and women with differing proclivities and in differing environments, times, and cultures. Yet in psychiatry, Falret, Kahlbaum, Kraepelin, and Bleuler maintained their attempts to apply Linnaean binomes to supposedly stereotyped deviations in behavior termed "mental diseases"—a conceptual atavism that W.F. Ogburn, Morris Cohen, and others have termed "cultural lag" in human thought. Adolf Meyer, one of the author's most revered teachers, proposed instead that we deal not with specific psychiatric afflictions but with interrelated effective or ineffective ways in which patients apply their energies, or, as Meyer termed them, their *ergasias* (from Greek, *ergon*, effort), in varied reactions to their stressful

47

milieu. Nevertheless, our current nosologic manuals [Third Edition of the DSM III in the U.S. (Appendix 1) or the Ninth International Classification of Diseases] still fail to distinguish mere psychiatric *nosology* (Gk.naming) or *taxonomy*[1] (Gk.listing) from a comprehensive clinical *diagnosis* (Gk. *discerning* knowledge) that would include significant constitutional and experiential factors, organic traumata, incidence of precipitating events, range of symptomatology, counterposed coping capacities and other important vectors that determine therapy and prognosis. Pressed by these considerations,[2] the APA Committee on Nomenclature added to their original formulations of DSM III the following "axes": I, the classified "disorder"; II, previous personality characteristics; III, contributory somatic diseases; IV, recent stresses; and V, the highest level of social functioning in the past year. True, if axes II through V were sufficiently developed during the examination and follow-up of the patient, they would lead beyond the always inadequate and often misleading nosologic label of Axis I to a thorough understanding of the patient's presenting and past difficulties and current potentialities. But even this is discouraged by an addendum (DSM III, p.24) that for Axis II only "a single personality [trait] will be noted," whereas Axes IV and V are to be limited to a "special clinical and research setting".

Other deficiencies of DSM III may be summarized as follows:

(1) *An Atavistic Nomenclature.* Examples: *Factitious* (false) *disorders, hypochondriasis* ("beneath the ribs" invalidism), *demoralization* (sinfulness?) and *borderline personality* (presuming there are lined boundaries between discrete "mental diseases"). Semantically misleading also are *mania* (Gk. spirit possession) and *melancholia* (excess of black bile), whereas *paranoia* (concepts other than the examiner's) and *schizophrenia* (split brain) are pejorataive labels that may have unjustifiably adverse social, actuarial and forensic effects on the patient.

(2) *A Lack of Cultural Relativity.* DSM III neglects to emphasize the almost infinite gradients of behavior from "normality" through "idiosyncratic," "neurotic" and "aberrant" to "psychotic" as differently regarded and treated in various contexts.[3]

(3) *Clinical and Scientific Cogency.* In general medicine, bare binomial designations (e.g., *mitral stenosis, diabetes mellitus*) are recognized as specifying almost nothing about the origin, pathophysiologic status, or extent and severity of bodily dysfunctions, let alone their comprehensive therapy. Instead, for an adequate diagnosis, adverse genetic, environmental, traumatic, toxic, infectious, and other pathogenic factors must be weighed against the patient's equally diverse sources of resistant, adaptive, and recuperative capacities. Such evaluations are essential in determining appropriate medical, environmental, and social therapies as influenced by economic, familial, ethnic, cultural, and other contingencies. Again, the ostensibly specific taxonomies of DSM III[4] obscure the highly variable vectors of constitutional and experiential etiology, age, intelligence, semeiology, cultural relevance, coping potentials and prognosis of the protean variations of "normal" and deviant behavior with which the clinician must deal, and thereby handicap comprehensive therapy and valid research.

**Empathetic Approaches to Diagnosis.** As indicated in Chapters 3 and 4, any retrospective survey of the vicissitudes of one's own life will recall periods of resentment, depression, alienation, and other, often excessive, responses to the stresses of our Western culture. These would include the poignant dependencies and separations of childhood, the questionings, rebellions and adventurous seekings of youth, the economic, sexual and cultural challenges of adulthood, the disillusioned reorientations and recastings of middle age, and the retrogressive longings of the later years (Chapter 14). By extension, we can better understand the more acute anxieties and their psychosomatic expressions of the "neurotic" when his modes of coping with physical, social, or metapsychologic uncertainties fail, resulting in obsessive preoccupations with, and compulsive avoidances (phobias) of symbolically threatening situations. When pressed down (depressed) too greatly by various Ur- frustrations, we, too reacted to some degree with loss of sleep, appetite, libido and *élan vitale*, and became dolorous, bitter and demandingly preemptive, or occasionally preoccupied with melancholy thoughts of surcease (and "revenge") through suicide. Conversely, we may have tried to rationalize our failures and aggrandize our status by attributing all our difficulties to the nefarious plots of envious enemies deliberately organized to contravene our righteousness and thwart our genius: steps toward grandiosity and "paranoia." And in our narcissistic reveries and dreams we have also, while immersed in strange affects, fancied ourselves independent of restraints of time, place, or logic, and masters of occult powers and esoteric consequences, hence we have differed from the schizophenic only in being less continuously divorced from a consensus of ambient "reality." Many of us have also had serious illnesses accompanied by delirious disorientation or even hallucinatory experiences before a return to rationality.

**Clinical Interrelationships.** In light of the above the following syndromes will be found more comprehensible in variable intensities and admixtures.

*Anxiety.* This is signaled by an unformulated but persistent apprehension expressed physically by cardiac palpitation, rapid, catchy respiration, pounding pulse, laryngeal spasms ("globus hystericus"), sweating, tremor, "flutterings in the stomach" (abdominal constrictions), urinary or colonic urgency, and other symptoms of psychosomatic imbalance. Often reported by the sufferer as "heart attacks," or "fainting spells," these episodes characteristically occur when the patient feels faced with harrowing doubts as to whether he can cope with serious threats to his physical, cultural, or philosophic securities: i.e., fears of disease or death (Ur I), of social isolation (Ur II), or of the erosion of cherished faiths (Ur III). Fortunately, such acute reactions also indicate latent vitality and mobility, so that helping the patient to clarify and dispel the source of his apprehensions may bring dramatic subjective and symptomatic relief.

*Phobic-Obsessive-Compulsive Syndromes.* These are characterized by persistent obsessions, fantasies, and fears (phobias) which, although recognized as partly irrational, nevertheless lead to rigidly patterned avoidances and stereotyped rituals

(compulsions). Typically, when these are frustrated, or interfered with even in therapy, the patient may react with anxiety or
anger (Chapter 15 or, Cases 1,3,4,5,6).

*Psychophysiologic Disturbances.* These comprise muscular
paralyses, mannerisms, tics, or other manifestations previously
termed hysterical (now "Briquet's syndrome"), accompanied either by excessive affect or with placid acceptance (*la belle indifference* if covertly satisfying to the patient). Psychogenic vago-
sympathetic imbalances may be expressed as mood-related
asthma, stress-induced spastic colitis, gastric spasms or ulcers,
urinary frequency, etc. (Chapter 15, Cases 2,8).

*Neuroses and "Borderline Personalities".* These are characterized by a protean variety of scholastic, sexual, marital, occupational, and cultural maladaptations; alcoholic and/or drug addictions; and covertly hostile or regressive patterns—all sufficiently
disapproved socially to render the patient uncomfortable, but
not yet subject to serious sanctions or legal confinement (Chapter 15, Case 12).

*Depressive Syndromes.* A typical semeiology includes the absence of appetite (*anorexia*, sometimes alternating with *bulimia*,
impulsive eating), variable constipation, insomnia or troubled
sleep, loss of weight, fatigability, hypochondriacal preoccupations, and sexual impotence or frigidity. Subjectively, there are
complaints of inability to concentrate, feelings of failure, guilt
and hopelessness and, in severe cases, melancholic ruminations
about death and suicide. Intermittent periods of forced, hollow
cheerfulness and restless, distracted overactivity (hypomania)
may occur, but are almost invariably succeeded by even deeper
depressive reactions. A patient with such manifestations is ex-
pressing desperate needs for concern and assistance, and if
these are not provided, he may suffer or die (by suicide) as
surely as one not given aid for a failing heart. Fortunately, most
*reactive depressions*, (i.e., precipitated by disabling physical, social,
or existential stresses) respond to mild sedatives, a protective milieu, and friendly, supportive therapeutic relationships that tide

the patient over critical periods and prevent tragic consequences. Deep *endogenous depressions* and those part of a possibly organic manic-depressive cycle require additional treatment with hormones, tricyclic drugs, lithium, electrotherapy and other measures, including hospitalization and suicide precautions (Chapters 6 to 15, Case 15).

*Pharmacotoxic States.* These result from taking excessive quantities of sedatives, tranquilizers, or stimulants, with resultant episodes of partial disorientation, sensory disturbances, confusions of thought and imagery, clouded memories or disinhibited sexual and aggressive behavior (cf. Chapter 15, Case 9). Conversely, sudden discontinuation or changes in drug intake may precipitate sensory derangements, muscular spasms, gastrointestinal dysfunctions, vague physiologic cravings, and other *withdrawal systems.* Especially in teen-age patients, inquiries must be made as to the excessive smoking of "pot" or "grass" (marijuana), the inhalation of volatile intoxicants (e.g., toluene or other commercial solvents in paints or adhesives), the consumption of "downers" (barbiturates) or "uppers" (amphetamines), or, even more dangerous individual or group experiments with lysergic acid, mescaline, quaalude, phencyclidine (angel dust) and other delirium-producing *psychotomimetic* substances. Irresponsible or naive parents may offer the euphemism "nervousness" as a cover for destructive, perverse, delinquent, or even delusional behavior in their intoxicated offspring (or mates), and may try to obtain yet more "tranquilizers" for them. Obviously, in such cases, a differential diagnosis is essential for proper therapy: the discontinuation of harmful drug intake, the control of withdrawal symptoms, and the correction of the rebellious and escapist behavior of which the patient's addiction to drugs may be but one manifestation.

*Paranoid States.* In these syndromes orientation to self, environment, and time is retained, but interpersonal relationships are distorted by false assumptions "logically" elaborated into convictions of being persecuted by a spreading cabal of conspirators; affects of anger and fear may accompany counterplotting and a compensatory grandiosity.

*Psychoses.* These become manifest when the patient's relationships to the therapist are grossly deviant, his sensorium confused, his thoughts illogical or bizarre, the concomitant affects manifestly inappropriate, the experiences he relates hallucinatory or indicative of delusions of persecution and grandeur, and his motivations uncontrolled and possibly dangerous. Just as it would be the physician's duty in the case of a reportable disease, it is here again the therapist's obligation to protect the patient and others by alerting his family and friends and by taking every measure, including legal steps, if necessary, to see that appropriate institutional care is secured (Chapter 15, Cases 11,12).

*Psychomotor Epilepsy or its Equivalents.* These comprise momentary suspensions of consciousness (*absences*) or confusional-amnesic states with or without local or generalized muscular twitches or transient "automatic" behavior (*fugues*), often followed by fatigue and headache. If the diagnosis is confirmed by direct observation supplemented by pathognomonic wave-forms on tracings of cerebral voltages (*electroencephalograms*), these episodes may be at least partially controlled by drugs such as phenobarbital, Tegrital, Dilantin, or Phenurone; or if persistent, in some cases by an operation on the cerebral or cerebellar cortex.

*Other Organic Impairments of Cerebral Function.* (Chapter 13). These may be due to the after effects of central nervous system infections, damages from concussion, hemorrhage, embolism or tumors, or the ravages of old age. Predictably, many patients who suspect grave and progressive impairments of their physical and intellectual powers will try to conceal or minimize serious symptoms such as localized headaches, visual and auditory impairment or recurrent episodes of confusion, and dismiss them as "just being overworked and a bit nervous." However, inquiry will reveal unmistakably progressive impairment of intellectual capacities and motor skills, loss of memory for recent events, and disintegration of personal and social habits.[5] Even when neurologic, opthalmoscopic, cerebrospinal fluid, roentgenologic findings confirm the diagnosis of focal or generalized cerebral lesions including the exceedingly debilitating effects of Alzheimer's disease (v. Appendix 2), the patient will all the more need reassurance, easing of strains and obligations, and guidance in utilizing his remaining capacities.

## Notes

1. Garrett Hardin comments (p.36) "A modern taxonomist must live with uncertainty or live falsely". And yet in a DSM III-related research based merely on mailed questionnaires processed by computers, the National Institute of Mental Health classified Americans as follows: 13.1 million suffered from anxiety disorders, 11.1 million from phobias, 10 million from substance abuse, 9.4 million from affective disorders, 2.4 million from obsessive-compulsive patterns, 1.6 million from "cognitive impairment" and 1.5 million from schizophrenia, constituting one-fifth of the total population.

2. By the author when he was President of the APA; and distinguished clinicians such as George Vaillant, Roy Menninger, John Spiegel and others.

3. Should Dukhobors whose religion demands an occasional nude public parade be arrested for obscenity? Are Catholics to be regarded as theopophagi for symbolically consuming flesh and blood at the Eucharist? Should Presbyterians who ecstatically "speak in tongues" (echolalia) or Holy Rollers who gyrate down church aisles or enter into bizarre trances after intense prayer be thought "schizoid"? Were the visions of Saints Bernadette or Joan of Arc, "schizophrenic"? Even apart from religious practices (which may also include catatonic stupors, self-immolation and mass homicide), is there any pattern of conduct in our culture that we regard as deviant that has not been accepted in other times or places as not only "normal" but highly commendable?

4. For a more detailed critique of DSM III, including the inadequacy of simple laboratory tests for complex behavior disorders, see B.J. Carroll, 1984.

5. According to Nobelist Roger Sperry, while the left cerebral hemisphere governs mathematics, spacial concepts, logic and other orientations to "reality" the right hemisphere deals with esthetics and empathetic social abstractions such as "love . . . mercy . . . beauty . . . courage . . . honor . . . justice . . ." difficult, if not impossible to formulate in arithmetical terms.

*Chapter 5*

# PREVIEW OF THE DYNAMICS
# OF THERAPY

### COMPARATIVE EXPERIMENTAL

During three decades of research in animal behavior[1] the author confirmed and extended the pioneer experiments of Ivan Pavlov, Howard Liddell, and Horsley Gantt in studies that led to the development of the following:

## Biodynamic Principles.

Principle *I, Motivation*: All animate behavior is actuated by physiologic needs for survival, procreation, and in higher animals, esthetic creativity.

Principle *II, Perception*: Every organism reacts not to an abstract "reality," but to its own interpretation of its milieu in terms of its unique capacities and experiences.

Principle *III, Adaptability*: When frustrated in pursuit of some satisfaction, organisms either modify their techniques or substitute their objectives to maintain an overall level of gratification.

Principle *IV, Neurotigenesis.* However, when simultaneous motivations are in sufficiently direct opposition so that the adaptive patterns required for each become mutually exclusive or conflictful, the organism experiences mounting uncertainty (anxiety), develops increasingly severe inhibitions, generalizing aversions (phobias), symbolic ritualizations (compulsions), muscular or organic (psychosomatic) dysfunctions, deviated social interactions (isolation, suspiciousness, sexual aberrations, excessive aggressivity or submissiveness) and other poorly adaptive neurotic behavior or aberrant and bizarre (psychotic) manifestations of hallucinations and delusions.

Principle *V, Therapy* The deviant responses outlined above can be alleviated by appropriate combinations of the following procedures in higher organisms:

### Experimental Therapies

(1)  Satisfaction of frustrated biologic needs
(2)  Change to a more favorable environment
(3)  Relief of uncertainties in adaptation
(4)  External pressure toward a tenable solution
(5)  Re-education by a trusted mentor (dyadic guidance)
(6)  Group influences
(7)  Alcohol or other nepenethic medications, with risk of addiction
(8)  Cerebral electroshock, with variable loss of skills
(9)  Limited operative lesions on the cerebral cortex, thalamus or hippocampus

These procedures in lower animals are analogous to the environmental, dyadic, group, medical and, if necessary, cerebrosurgical modalities employed in clinical therapy (Chapters 5 to 15). However, since human beings are endowed, or burdened, with a far greater range of perceptions, interpretations, and potentials for action, clinical therapy requires correspondingly greater degrees of comprehension and skill as outlined below.

## Essential Modalities of Clinical Therapies[2]

Perhaps the most regrettable source of public confusion about psychiatry is the multiplicity of treatments advocated, many by nonpsychiatrists, for various behavior disorders. Under one or another esoteric designation, differing "schools" and cults present claims and counterclaims, but few offer a tenable rationale or cite adequately controlled results. Therefore, during my presidency of the American Psychiatric Association from 1978 to 1979, I appointed six authorities[3] in the field to constitute a Commission on Therapies charged with the following tasks:

(1)   To assay as many as possible of the somatic, environmental, dyadic, group, familial, and social modes of treatment in current use (a) by gathering additional data from previous APA reports, (b) by a thorough and critical examination of the literature on techniques, duration, results, costs, and other characteristics, (c) by direct consultations with advocates of differing modalities and (d) by direct observation of various treatments where practicable, or through viewing of videotapes, questionnaires and other means;

(2)   To analyze the findings as to common therapeutic vectors, as distinguished from procedures that may be extraneous or counterproductive;

(3)   To prepare a series of reports to be coordinated, edited, and published by the APA.

In the following 5 years, in accord with its charge, the Commission reviewed and abstracted an extensive library of books and articles, interviewed or received manuscripts from hundreds of consultants, held numerous meetings with the author, submitted interim reports, edited and re-edited them, and finally integrated them in a 908 page volume under the comprehensive title *The Psychiatric Therapies*, published by the APA Press in 1984. Herewith a summary of my final chapter on the basic dynamics of the several hundred modalities of therapy reviewed in that volume.

## THE ESSENTIAL DYNAMICS OF THERAPY[4]

**(1) The Reputation of the Therapist** (merited or illusory). The anticipatory confidence of a patient in an individual therapist (as derived from his academic position, scientific or popular writings, commendable public appearances, and most of all by favorable reports from colleagues and current or former patients) plays an important initial role in all therapies. The patient's wishful expectancy of cure, whether by thaumaturgy, primal scream, dream analysis, or divine intervention, constitutes a powerful preliminary advantage to the prospective therapist, be he faith healer, neuropsychiatrist, psychoanalyst, or priest.

**(2) Rapport** (productive or seductive). This consists essentially of trust on the part of the patient that the therapist will meet one or more of the patient's triune (Ur) needs, i.e. when:

He *fears* that his physical welfare and bodily skills are threatened by disease, trauma, or deterioration, or that

His familial, sexual, or social interrelationships *appear* to be failing, or when

His cherished convictions (i.e., rationalized or mystically wishful beliefs)[5] *seem* no longer a source of adequate comfort.

The patient's trepidations are paraphrased *subjectively* (i.e., "fear," "appear," "seem") to emphasize that his *concepts* of his current or impending difficulties (e.g., "I'm afraid my pains mean cancer," "My neighbors plan to burn my house," or "I am going to hell for what I've done") imbue his appeals for help, irrespective of "objective" evaluations of his physical state, social status, or ultimate fate. The therapist should therefore appear competent in all three therapeutic roles:

As a physician (nurse, physical-therapist, et al.) well trained
to diagnose and treat somatic ills.

As a friend (social worker, marital counsellor) whose empathy indicates to the patient that he may have found an ally in an otherwise unpredictable or hostile world.

And as a seer and mentor who can help resolve existential dilemmas.

**(3) Relief** (rational or escapist). Two principle modes for this are open:

(a) As a physician, the therapist should, as indicated, utilize every available skill he/she possesses to relieve actual or anticipated pain, distress, or dysfunction. If urgent for states of agitation or desperation, sodium amytal may be administered intravenously. Subsequent medications, with due precautions as to incompatibilities, overdoses, plasma levels, and addictions may include the benzodiazepines for tension, a mild flurazepam for insomnia, a tricyclic or one of the newer drugs for depression, carefully monitored lithium for manic hyperactivity and the phenothiazines, or butyrophenones for schizophrenic behavior (Chapter 12). (b) Concurrently, amelioration of environmental stresses may consist of relief from detested work, incompatible associates, or an intolerable milieu or, if necessary, day, night, or continuous hospitalization.

**(4) Review** (objective or preconceived). With somatic distress partially alleviated, the grateful patient, under gentle and tactful but skillfully directed inquiry (Chapter 3), will be more willing to consider the real or imagined circumstances that precipitated his other current dysfunctions, which will almost never correspond to any stereotyped diagnostic category (Chapter 4 and Appendix 1). A truly comprehensive survey of the patient's familial, educational, sexual, social, occupational, marital, and related experiences should reveal not only his physical and psychologic vulnerabilities, but also prognostically relevant talents and assets (Chapter 5). Confessions of past or current misconduct may be therapeutic not because of any inherent "cathartic" or "abreactive" effect but insofar as they are received by a reassuringly sympathetic and helpful therapist.

**(5) Reconsideration and Reorientation** (realistic or solipsistic). During the patient's accounts of early or recent experiences (irrespective of his or her position on a chair or couch, in a supine or lotus position, whether in dyadic or group interchanges, or in brief, prolonged, few, or multiple sessions) the therapist, with or without group surrogates, through verbal or other modes of communication, explores the patient's concepts, symbolisms, values and conduct, and explicitly or implicitly conveys effective clarifications and re-evaluations. These interchanges, if skillfully conducted, lead the patient to reconsider whether, even at the price of surrendering his formerly cherished dependent, seductive, aggressive, vengeful, or other covert gratifications, alterations in his patterns of conduct would on the whole bring more substantial and lasting physical, social, and metapsychologic rewards.

**(6) Resocialization** (inclusive or restricted). This consists of the patient applying the reorientations acquired as above to more adequately adaptive familial, occupational, social, esthetic, cultural, and creative conduct: first in his individual or group sessions, and concurrently or eventually outside the office, clinic, retreat, or hospital—thereby demonstrating true operational e-motional," (literally, "to move out") rather than "intellectual" (i.e., merely verbal) insight.

**(7) Recycling** (progressive or retrogressive). Finally, as in any other form of re-education, it is often necessary to re-establish faltering rapport, relieve recrudescences of symptoms, refurbish previous understandings, reconsider remaining departures from rational conduct, and repeat portions of the process as often as necessary until stability is restored.

### NOTES

1.  Masserman, J.H. *The Biodynamic Roots of Human Behavior*, 1968; my chapter on Biodynamics in Kaplan, Freedman, & Sadock, *Comprehensive Textbook of Psychiatry*, Williams & Wilkins, 3rd ed., 1980, pp. 782-790; and research films (v. Bibliography).

2.  P. London had characterized psychotherapy as "an ill-defined technique applied to an unknown population with indeterminate results; for this, long and arduous training is required."

3.  Seymour Malleck, MD, Byram Karasu, MD, Stanley Lesse, MD, Judd Marmor, MD, John Nemiah, MD, and Nicholas Cummings, PhD, President of the American Psychological Association.

4.  Whimsically, since there are seven parameters and all begin with the letter R, they were dubbed, to paraphrase T.E. Lawrence, the Seven Pil-R's of Therapeutic Wisdom.

5.  The patient's needs may include a suitable form of immortality, i.e.: "The American Indians looked forward to their happy hunting ground. The Norsemen expected to go to a place where there was war all day long, but in the evening all wounds were healed [so that fighting could resume next morning]. The Mohammedans looked forward to a place of sensuous delight featuring wine, women, and song. The Christians anticipate a heaven of golden streets and the music of harps. The Jews hope for an Academy on High, where God joins with the faithful in ceaseless study. . .When missionaries approached the Eskimos and told them of the heat of hell. . . anything suggestive of warmth appealed to them." (Phillip Waterman, p.275). Such hopes need never be challenged in therapy.

# Chapter 6

# INTRODUCTION TO THERAPY

Guided by the preliminary interviews (Chapter 3), the therapist will proceed in his triple (Ur) functions as physician, social counsellor, and philosophic mentor, shunning the extremes of impassive observer, cultural agnostic, or ethical pontiff. With respect for the patient's unique expectations, intelligence, and initial receptivities, the following explanations at appropriate times will clarify and expedite therapy.

**Procedures.** Most dyadic therapies can be conducted with the patient and therapist comfortably seated facing each other. Alternatively, the patient may be placed on a couch as an aid to relaxation, as facilitating spontaneous expressions, as relieving him from scrutinizing and possibly misjudging the therapist's reactions, or as enhancing a therapeutic and not merely a conversational setting.

**Medical Measures.** Physical and neurologic examinations and laboratory tests are conducted and medications prescribed if needed for sleep, abstention from alcohol, dietary deficiencies, intercurrent symptoms or other medical reasons (Chapter

13). Ancillary diagnostic and therapeutic procedures such as hypnosis (Chapter 7) or sodium amytal (Chapter 12) will be utilized if helpful, but only after thorough explanations and the patient's well informed consent.

**Communication.** The patient is invited to express his thoughts, fantasies, desires, and affects without inhibition. He is also assured that his feelings about the therapist will not be taken personally, but as reflections of former or current attitudes toward other important persons in his life. (Chapter 8)

**Confidentiality.** All communications will be held privileged. Notes may be taken, but will be available to no one other than the therapist or an agreed-upon consultant. The patient is also advised to keep his experiences in therapy largely to himself to avoid extramural misunderstandings.

## RESPONSIBILITY

As soon as tactfully possible it should be made clear that since the world at large will hold the patient accountable for his behavior, therapy will proceed on that basis. This could apply even to involuntary behavior, such as epileptic seizures or dyskinesias, since what the patient does to prevent or ameliorate them is still within his purview.

**Motivations.** Every person is primarily concerned with what he *conceives* to be his own welfare, the significant differences then being in whether his conduct is ultimately profitable or, though temporarily gratifying, eventually disadvantageous. Such formulations are in no sense cynical: a war hero, an obscure scientist, or an anonymous philanthropist may each render invaluable public services even though the hero may be envisaging public accolade, the scientist academic advancement or the Nobel Prize, and the philanthropist angelic wings and canonization.

**Conative Clarification.** If an alcoholic protests "If I didn't want to stop drinking I wouldn't be coming to therapy," it may be pointed out that he would indeed like to be rid of his headaches, tremors, gastric ulcer, and his wife's and employer's warnings, but that his desires to drink obviously override all contrary considerations. Since he refuses Antabuse, hospitalization, or other recommended measures, the issue is not *whether*, but really *why* he wishes to continue drinking—i.e., as an escape from reality, defiance of authority, covert desires to be fired or divorced, disinhibition of aggressive or erotic conduct, regression to helplessness with misleading appeals for succor, or other such covert gratifications. Until he uncovers and surrenders these objectives and cultivates others more socially adaptable, he may well continue his alcoholic indulgences despite the physical and social penalties involved while rationalizing that he cannot control his genetically preordained "disease of alcoholism" (Chapter 13).

**Centrality.** In other subtle denials of responsibility, patients will speak in terms such as, "The thought came to me that. . ." "A mood overcame me to. . ." "My rage (or other emotion) made me do. . ." or in similar language implying helplessness rather than choice. The therapist may inquire as to just how the thought or mood, if not his own, came: by radar, telepathy, or parcel post? And, does not "e-motion" mean how one *chooses* to "move out?"

**Directiveness.** The therapist will not—indeed, cannot— direct or control the patient's behavior other than to make as clear as possible his motivations, his past maladaptive patterns, and alternative options that the patient may then explore and adopt as ultimately more socially acceptable and rewarding. However, there is one important exception to which the patient must agree: in case of premonitions of homicidal, suicidal, or other desperate acts, the therapist reserves an option to take whatever course, in collaboration with whomever he thinks best, to prevent such catastrophes (Chapter 13). His action will be as minimally revelatory of the patient as possible, but this eventuality, however rare, must be anticipated in the best interests of all concerned.

## PRECONCEPTIONS

Among complicating notions with which many patients come to therapy are these:

**Childhood Engrams.** A patient may avidly wish to believe that his current behavior stems inevitably from having been neglected, rejected, seduced, overworked, overindulged, or otherwise improperly treated early in life. Ergo, he will blame his parents, siblings, teachers, et al. and not himself for his deviant behavior on the plea that his "childhood traumata" had left adverse and irremediable effects. Such rationalizations may be met by tactfully phrased counterploys to the effect that he has since had many opportunities to moderate his rebellions, escapisms, and other counterproductive reactions, and to respond cooperatively to more friendly environments had he really wished to do so—and can do so now.

**Sexuality.** From readings in early Freud or other monothetic literature, some patients, especially those with marital or extramarital difficulties, may insist that their troubles are directly attributable to basic "sexual maladjustments." True, sex other than masturbation is an interpersonal event, but its significance lies not in its modality, frequency, or object, but whether it is employed for mutually friendly intercourse, or for self-assurance, seduction, escape, dependence, conquest, dominance, or similar counterproductive purposes (Chapter 14).

**Dreams, Fantasies, Ruminations.** Also from psychoanalytic readings, patients will inquire whether they should remember and relate their dreams "as the royal road to the unconscious." Explanations of their relevance may take the following form: were the patient to daydream that he won the Nobel Prize in Literature, his motivations at the moment would be obviously different than if he were fantasizing a liaison with a cinema actress (or hero), picturing the humiliation of a hated rival, or visualizing the beneficent testament of a dying relative. Similarly, dreams may be obviously or covertly indicative of the dreamer's wishes, and even nightmares may explore symbolically feared situations so that one can awaken to comparative security. Ergo, if the patient considers a dream somehow significant, he should relate it at the next session; however, excessive preoccupation with dreams and fantasies may be an attempt to induce the therapist to join the patient in diversions from waking reality, and will be considered as such.

## RESISTANCES

At some favorable opportunity during the initial interviews the patient may be confronted with the fact that while many persons are willing to pay handsomely for frequent sessions of rationalized baby-sitting, no one really likes the disillusioning and often wrenching reorientations and readaptations of effective psychiatric therapy. By analogy, patients apply to dentists or surgeons to relieve a toothache or be rid of a cancer, yet few enjoy being drilled or operated upon *per se*. So also in psychotherapy: despite the patient's discomfort over the adverse physical and social consequences of his deviant behavior, resistances to re-exploring and altering long-cherished patterns of thought and action may take various obvious or covert forms, among them:

(a) "Forgetting," coming late, or cancelling appointments. If, however, the patient is ill, has a truly important conflicting obligation, or has other valid reasons for the cancellation, he should not be thought "resistant" or charged for the missed interview, since this would impair the reality-oriented aspects of the therapy.

(b) Deciding after a few sessions that the therapist has effected a wondrous cure and that treatment can be terminated. Again, by analogy, a dentist may rapidly relieve pain, but knows —and must so inform the patient—that a residual abscess will continue to be toxic and destructive unless more deeply and thoroughly treated. So also, in psychotherapy, the patient will be invited to continue for a few sessions either to resolve remaining difficulties or to confirm that there has been a really stable "flight into health."

As a variant, the patient may decide that some fantastic scheme will resolve all his troubles. A patient might propose to divorce his wife, quit his career as a symphony player, move to Alaska and open a mink farm with an utterly charming waitress he had met the preceding week—with thanks to the therapist for helping free the patient from his "former shackles." It is important to anticipate such impulses to escape from therapy (and reality) by stating that while the therapist could not ethically interfere with the patient's behavior short of preventing homicide or suicide, it would be best to consider drastic changes in his life thoroughly in therapy before embarking on courses he might eventually regret.

## FREQUENCY, DURATION, AND COST OF THERAPY

The patient's questions in these regards, direct or implicit, should be answered as frankly and explicitly as possible. The optimum frequency of therapeutic sessions may range from a single interview to five times weekly, or to intermittent or continuous hospitalization. However, since the duration of therapy is contingent on many considerations, the following or a similar analogy may be employed. If a cello teacher is asked how long it would take for a student to improve his playing, the teacher could reply only that it would depend on the student's talents, how often and effectively he practices to correct deficiencies in musical perception, technique, and expression as revealed in his lessons, how harmoniously he begins to coordinate his playing with others in a chamber ensemble or symphony orchestra, how closely he wishes ultimately to approach virtuosity, or, in the case of pedagogues, how well he could teach others. So also, even with the best of therapy, what the patient achieves in what length of time will depend more on his receptivity for understanding and his goals for individual improvement and social concordance, than solely on the therapist's skill and guidance.

As to the estimated cost of the treatment, the therapist may point out that, since each session, for optimum benefit, may last forty or more minutes, he is as a specialist justified in charging considerably more than a general practitioner's usual fee. However, although in many instances the average total expense of therapy would be less, say, than the cost of an appendectomy, the actual amount would again depend on the rapidity of the patient's progress, which the therapist could expedite only insofar as the patient permits. As to the method of compensation, daily mercenary transactions can be avoided by having the therapist's secretary mail monthly statements of amounts due, which the patient is expected to pay in full. If, however, even this causes the patient unnecessary hardship, the issue can be discussed in therapy and there resolved.

## SEMANTICS

Especially in the beginning phases of therapy, patients will use words and phrases that are supposed to convey explicit meanings, yet are either so vague, evasive, or inclusive as to require operational clarification. Examples:

**Reticence.** If, when spontaneous communications are requested, the patient states, "I am not thinking of anything" he denies the fact that everyone thinks continuously every waking (and probably sleeping as well as dreaming) moment. The statement merely conveys a desire not to reveal troublesome ideas, possibly because of their unwelcome significance.

**Innocence through Ignorance.** "I can't remember what [people say] I did" . . . or "why I did it." To which it may be pointed out that the patient was probably not in a coma at the time, that he alone knows best not only what he did but implicitly also why he did it, that at this moment in therapy he apparently would rather not explore his motivations, but that eventually he will understand and perhaps modify them to his advantage.

**"Habits," "Compulsions," "Irresistible Impulses," etc..** It may also be pointed out that these are rationalized terms for modes of behavior in which a person persists only as long as he finds them gratifying, and which he can therefore change whenever he so desires. For example, a 30-year overindulgence in tobacco or alcohol can be stopped at any time a person finally becomes sufficiently concerned about a bloody cough, or a jail sentence for drunken driving.

**"Love".** With this four-letter word a patient may cover attitudes that range from marginal attraction to an object or person that offers moderate physical, social, or imagined satisfactions, to stronger affection when the possible rewards seem major, to infatuation when one expects the fulfillments to be maximal.

**"Hate".** Refers to the obverse of the above, ranging from mild aversions to objects or people who might minimally disappoint to homicidal wishes against those regarded as unbearably frustrating.

**"Guilt".** By using this term the patient invites commendation for his conscientious remorse over some thought or deed for which he basically fears punishment on earth or in some later purgatory.

**Jargon.** From classes or readings[1] in abnormal (sic) psychology or from previous therapists, the patient may have acquired a vocabulary of "id impulses," "complexes," anal or oral "fixations," "ego defenses," "identity crises," and other such pseudoerudite patois. Without denigrating former teachers or therapists who may have cherished them, such verbal ambiguities should be translated into recognizable desires, doubts, interpersonal attachments or other more meaningful concepts. Reciprocally, the therapist should use direct and clear language in commenting on the patient's communications and behavior in the session as well as on his reports of his attitudes and conduct elsewhere. Easily misconstrued jargon should be avoided: e.g., "naracissistic" for exclusively self-centered; "neurosis" for a pattern of counterproductive idiosyncrasies; "cathexes" for motivationally charged; "introjects" for persons dead or alive with whom the patient continues to be symbolically involved; "masochism" for milder expiatory suffering to gain sympathy and avoid greater punishment; "soul" for a mystical disembodiment; "existential," usually regarded by most patients as about as meaningful as Gertrude Stein's "a rose is a rose is a rose"; or the "Self," conceptually capitalized (as deified) and misapplied operationally (L. Wittgenstein). Although euphemistically seductive, such terms have little place in pragmatic therapy.

**Duplicity.** "I keep telling myself to (or not to . . .)," "I find myself . . .," "I hate myself," etc., are expressions in which the patient wishes to picture a virtuous and praiseworthy *I* with whom he identifies, but who, unfortunately, is perverted and martyred by a disowned *myself*, over which the commendable *I* has little or no control. The therapist should again help the patient recognize that even if a few obtuse listeners temporarily accept this "double personality" pretense, society will eventually punish the deeds of his "myself" so that, unfortunately, his "I" will concurrently suffer. Other portentously vacuous pronouncements may be similarly met with various combinations of tact and incisiveness: "I want to be myself!" (Who else are you now?); "I want to be able to communicate better" (What to whom?); "I long to (have a right to) be free!" (From what? whom? all restraints?); "I hate myself!" (plan to sue?).

**Recycling** (Chapter 5). The therapist can be almost certain that all of his preliminary explanations, clarifications, arrangements, cautions, etc., will be "forgotten," misconstrued, or flouted during subsequent therapy. However, their repetition during relevantly crucial periods will be all the more effective if they have been explained during early interviews.

### COUPLES, FAMILY, AND GROUP SESSIONS

Again in a manner appropriate to the personnel and the occasion, participants should be made generally aware of the issues briefed above, with further emphasis on the following:

That the gathering is in no sense an arbitration or judicial hearing to determine who among them is "right" or "wrong," "normal," or "neurotic," but rather an occasion for the airing of individual thoughts, feelings, and concerns for mutual under-standings and helpful applications. The therapist will be a per-ceptive, empathetic, nonpartisan monitor devoted to the welfare of all concerned. As such, he will function to give everyone an opportunity for participation and interaction but may, if neces-sary, request that overly strident accusations, violent quarrels, or other counterproductive behavior be contained.

At the end of one or several sessions, the therapist may sug-gest that one or more of the participants return for personal in-terviews or counseling, provided that he or she will concentrate on his or her own conduct rather than solely on complaints of mistreatment by others. As a trenchant analogy: a musical en-semble cannot play harmoniously unless each member plays his own instrument and part well, rather than claim that all the oth-ers are out of time and tune.

## TERMINATION OF THERAPY

This should usually occur when both the patient(s) and the therapist agree that the former has achieved adequate physical well-being, social adaptations, and psychologic ("Ur") serenity, or that these objectives will progress to satisfactory levels without further intensive therapy, with only occasional follow-ups, or with renewals only if special needs or crises should recur. Pa-tients, though cautioned as above, are of course privileged to terminate at any time; but so also is the therapist if he feels that they merely continue in a dependent, escapist role and wish to make no further accountable progress.

## NOTE

1. For similar reasons, the patient may be cautioned that articles on psychology and psychiatry in popular magazines or paper-backs may furnish misleading information, whereas, if the pa-tient consults professional works on these subjects (including the author's) he may misconstrue the text and misapply it to himself.

*Chapter 7*

# HYPNOSIS

Perhaps the most vivid illustration of direct therapist-patient interaction is furnished by a syndrome first called by Anton Mesmer (1734–1815) "animal magnetism" and by James Braid (1795–1860) "hypnotism" (Gk. *hypnnos*, sleep). Both terms are misleading, since what is currently termed hypnosis connotes a state in which a subject, independent of physical influences and with or without "sleep" or "trance," merely consents for a limited time to speak or act in some ways acceptable to him as suggested by the hypnotist.

## SUSCEPTIBILITY

In view of the above, everyone is in some sense "hypnotizable," to a degree of compliance that can then be roughly measured by various preliminary tests. These range from assertions that the intertwined fingers of two hands cannot be pulled apart (a normally surmountable result of induced tensions), to the obvious subservience of a subject who, after spreading his legs, sways to a suggested side, or backward, when the back of his head is touched by the hypnotist.

## TECHNIQUE OF INDUCTION

**1. Physical.** The subject rests on a comfortable chair or couch in a quiet room free of distractions, and is reassured as to the somatic and psychologic benefits of the projected hypnosis. He is then requested to concentrate on rhythmic tones or lights, preferably synchronous with his pulse, to induce a state of progressive relaxation and somnolence while remaining in sole communication with the hypnotist.

### 2. Interpersonal

*(a) Maternal Soothing.* With or without the above sensory counterpoint, the hypnotist, in cadences reminiscent of a lullaby, suggests that various portions of the patient's body feel progressively more "comfortable . . . relaxed . . . at ease . . . warm . . . tingling . . . floating . . . ," leading to a persuasive "You will close your eyes . . . you will become more and more drowsy . . . drowsy . . . drowsy . . . sleepy . . . sleepy . . . as I count slowly from 1 to 10 you will become more and more relaxed . . . drowsy . . . sleepy . . . (a misleading but effective term) . . . 1 . . . 2 . . . 3 . . . 4 . . . 10! . . . now you must sleep . . . deeply . . . deeply . . . you cannot open your eyes . . . you cannot wake . . . you can hear only my voice . . . you will follow my suggestions . . . and do as I say . . . " (Here compliance may be tested by insensitivity to a mild pinprick, holding an arm rigid, etc.—although the subject will either break collaboration if ordered to act in any way unacceptable to him or her, or assert later that it was done under compulsion.) Hypnosis may usually be terminated by "Now that you are relaxed . . . rested . . . I will let you awake as I count slowly backward from 10 . . . to 1! You will wake refreshed . . . relaxed of your (symptom) . . . and happy to do as I suggested" (if posthypnotic directives are to be employed with or without conscious recall of the corresponding hypnotic experience).

*(b) Paternal Authoritative.* In this modality—usually employed by stage hypnotists or practiced on especially subservient subjects—the technique consists of imperious gestures and commands to "Sleep! . . . you cannot open your eyes . . . there is no

one here but me . . . you must do as I say until I wake you . . . and without remembering why." Here also "posthypnotic amnesia" may be professed, but is easily penetrable.

**3. Mystic.** This third mode of induction employs lush draperies, a quasi-thaumaturgic atmosphere, shining crystal balls or kaleidoscopic lights, magic gestures by the hypnotist, and other impressively occult bewitchings.

Any combination of these procedures may indeed induce a state of intensive attention and rapport in which the "hypnotized" subject may obligingly produce previously repressed memories,[1] agree to surrender progressively unwanted symptoms or behavior patterns, and awake on signal feeling refreshed and grateful. However, at no time was the hypnozand really "asleep" or in a mystic "trance," nor could he or she be compelled to perform then or later acts incompatible with his or her personal or social principles. Although these may be sufficiently lax to permit conduct contrary to moral or legal standards, the hypnotist may later be blamed for these aberrations, and berated or sued accordingly.

### EVALUATION[2]

Because of its aura of thaumaturgic control, hypnosis is perennially appealing to eager therapists who may combine it with drugs (H. Spiegel), pseudoanalytic "interpretations" (J. Rosen), and even regressions to "intrauterine experiences and rebirth" (R. Hubbard). The drawbacks of hypnosis are not that patients become submissive to the will of the therapist; even in fiction Trilby repeatedly defied Svengali when it suited her to do so. The difficulties are that some therapists become wishfully misled as to the interpersonal dynamics and limitations of hypnosis, and therefore do not reserve its use to precisely appropriate times with carefully selected patients who are ready for favorable changes in behavior in a more comprehensive therapeutic program. Otherwise the effects of hypnosis are short-lived and complications of disappointment, suspicion, resentment, and even paranoid delusions of influence and seduction may occur.

Hyppolyte Bernheim, a thorough student of hypnosis who taught Freud, offered two aphorisms: "It is a wise hypnotist who knows who is hypnotizing whom," and "There is little that can be done with hypnosis that cannot be done better, and with fewer complications without it." (Chapter 15, Case 11)

## NOTES

1.  The author's final disillusionment with so-called "hypnotic regressions" occurred when a compliant patient described not only the precise details of her second birthday party, but also "remembered" her experiences at birth and her preceding fourth intrauterine month—imprints neurophysiologically impossible for an unmyelinated neonatal, let alone an embryonic brain. For such reasons, testimony obtained under hypnosis is inadmissible in most courts of law.

2.  For a detailed discussion of hypnotic facts and fallacies, v. Masserman, 1955, pp.585-594.

*Chapter 8*

# PSYCHOANALYSES

## THEORIES AND THERAPIES IN MODERN DYNAMIC TERMS

In 1909, G. Stanley Hall, founder of the American Psychological Association, invited Sigmund Freud, Carl Jung and five of their disciples to lecture on psychoanalysis at Clarke University. William James, Charles Pierce, John Dewey and other leading American scholars who were present evaluated the presentations adversely; however, their unique analytic advocacy of therapeutic libidinal freedom in a repressive age, followed by Henry Brill's translation of Freud's *Interpretation of Dreams* and *Studies of Hysteria* intrigued many clinicians previously bound by genetic and nihilistic concepts of sexual aberrations, "neuroses," "psychasthenias" and related disorders. Psychoanalytic Insitutes were founded in New York, Chicago and elsewhere, and began to train students in an increasingly rigid curriculum: reading all of Freud's writings and those of his loyal disciples, a personal analysis lasting for years, supervised analytic therapy of four or more assigned patients, and strictly monitored adherence to classical doctrines and practices before admission to an official Psychoanalytic Society. On this basis psychoanalysts acquired so initially dazzling an aura of esoteric wisdom that they were long considered an elite among therapists, while others often claimed to base their therapy "on psychoanalytic principles."

This chapter will review sometimes conflicting aspects of "classical" and modern psychoanalysis (a) as a form of research, (b) as a theory of behavior, (c) as a technique of treatment and (d) as interpretations of anthropology, sociology, biology, esthetics, and futurology.

## PSYCHOANALYTIC CONCEPTS

**Libido.** This now ubiquitous term was first equated primarily with the sexual drive, but has since acquired other quasierotic connotations as follows:

*Primary Narcissism.* Self-love, according to Freud, is first expressed in the infant's *"polymorphous delight"* in discovering various parts and functions of its own body. Objects with which the infant interacts are then invested ("cathected") with *secondary narcissism*, eventually extended to the *"introjection"* of significant personages as also parts of the *narcissistic self*. Illusions of solipsistic dominance spring from the subservience of such personages summoned by the cry of the child, and are later reflected in the magic of the Voice and the Word; in dreams of independence of space and time, or in the delusions of the paranoic or schizophrenic.

*Birth Trauma.* In certain early analytic theories much was made of the concept that the first serious threat to the life of an organism occurs when it leaves the absolute security of the womb and is born precariously into the blaring, threatening confusion of the outside world. According to Rank (and Kierkegaard and others before him), this constitutes the root of all subsequent anxiety, and the consequent longings of all mankind for a return to a quasi-prenatal "Nirvana"—not in the Hindu concept of *non*-being but, as presented in other religions as an all-provident, peaceful, and secure existence.

*Oral Incorporation.*   The infant, usually in its mother's arms,[1] also senses that its lips, mouth, and tongue are the organs by which it obtains satisfaction of its essential nutritive needs, as later displaced kinesthetically to pacifier, or thumb, pipe stems, or the unlit cigar. Oral erotism is also expressed in various sexual activities ranging from kissing—"normal" in many societies—to various "oral perversions" acceptable publicly in relatively few. Counter-reactions range from the compensatory oral engorgements of neurotic *bulimia*, to the delusion of "having swallowed the world" of the schizophrenic. So, too, may arise the mystic rites of the incorporation of the beneficent god common to many religions.

*Oral Aggressivity.*   However, when earlier incorporative satisfactions become frustrated, the infant reacts with possessive or vengeful behavior, seen during weaning in active chewing of the nipple, reflected later in various verbal or gestural patterns such as "biting saracasm" or gnashing the teeth during frustrated rage. Conflicts between passive oral longings and reactive hostilities also appear in hyperpeptic and hyperacidic gastric disorders and in *anorexia nervosa*, in which the self-starvation and protracted vomiting to deny the destructive symbolism of eating may become so severe as to endanger the life of the patient.[2]

*Anal Erotism.*   Later, the human infant becomes concerned with another body function which gives repeated "pleasure" through recurrent physiological relief; namely, the evacuation of the bowels and bladder. It is a common pediatric observation that infants have no aversion for their metabolic products; on the contrary, unrestricted children may play with or eat their feces. This period of "treasuring" the body products is known as the *anal rententive* phase of development. In later life, *anal eroticism* may remain as a hidden component in many personal and cultural patterns such as the quasi-masturbatory seclusiveness of the excretory act, an obsession that "regular bowel movements" are essential to health, and anal sexual perversions.

*Anal Aggression.*   Somewhat later in the infant's life he faces the necessity of making his first serious social adaptation—that of controlling his bowel movements until the proper place and time for evacuation. To the parent this training appears to be but a part of "natural development," but to the child it may be a time of libidinal inhibitions and reorientations as sweeping and as difficult as any he may, with far greater resources, be called on to make in later life. For he is no longer the autonomous ruler of parents who had previously satisfied almost every want. Rather, the parents now turn into ever more firm taskmasters. This readjustment is a stressful one; should bowel training and other disciplines be started too early or be too harsh and abrupt, *anal aggressiveness* may be expressed in the infant and child by "mischievous" self-indulgence in dirt and filth, combined with destructive habits of soiling, breaking, and scattering. Similarly, the adult may delight in scatologic jokes and expressions, adhere to mud-baths or similar mysophilic pursuits, or fetishistic pleasure in accumulating and hoarding "filthy lucre." Conversely, a patient may become so fearful of contamination by "dirt" that most of his waking life is spent in rituals of washing, cleaning, and sterilizing so that he might not befoul himself or others and, in either case, be quasi-parentally punished.

*Genital Erotism.* Penile and clitoral erections in human infants occur in the first months of life, and their detumescence on manipulation is accompanied by unmistakable relief of restlessness—a fact utilized by pragmatic nursemaids. Susan Isaacs has also described voyeuristic, exhibitionistic, and other "phallic" activities in children only two years old. Halverson (1940) observed that genital erections in infants aged three to twenty weeks occur in apparent compensations for oral or anal frustrations. Masturbation with partial orgasm may begin in the first year and continue irregularly thereafter in both sexes. Heterosexual fantasies are later derived from observing sexual differences in parents, siblings, and other children, from witnessing coitus between parents (the *primal scene*), and from exploring heterosexual contacts, as yet only rarely associated with concepts of impregnation or childbirth.

The persons about whom early sexual fantasies revolve are usually those within the family. In the case of the boy, it is his mother or an older sister; in the girl, sexual erotism is also directed toward the mother and only later transferred toward the father or some male surrogate. But the boy and the girl have observed that the mother, however much they may desire her exclusively, really belongs to the father who remains in the parental bed and retains the right to demand and obtain her sexual attentions. Thus, according to "classical" analytic theory, children of both sexes experience the so-called *Oedipus complex*, more comprehensively discussed in Chapter 2. But in the case of most children the Laius analogy does not hold, since the all-powerful father, instead of being displaced, remains very much alive and quite capable of depriving the child of the organic nidus of its fantasies of maternal erotic possession. In the case of the boy, this *castration fear* may have diverse determinants: the association of erotic wishes with his erectile penis, threats of castration made to deter the child's masturbation, or observations of the genitalia of girls and women who appear to have been actually castrated. Thus genitality may become charged with persistent *guilts* (unconscious apprehensions of punishment) that color all the later patterns of personal and social behavior. Masturbation with incest fantasies is thus feared as leading not only to loss of "manhood" or "womanhood," but also to disease and insanity. Or, in his interpersonal contacts, the adult with a deeply ingrained *incest guilt* may either abjure heterosexual contacts, or lead a sex life of loveless, restless promiscuity (*Don Juanism* in men, *nymphomania* in women), or become reactively aggressive toward either sex, or fly from heterosexuality altogether either into precarious homosexual relationships or regressive asexual dependencies.

*Postoedipal Development: The latent period.*[3]   In orthodox analytic theory it was thought that after the ages of five or six years, erotic libidinal tensions abated and became relatively quiescent until puberty, at which time the maturation of the gonads reawakened psychosexuality. However, many child analysts (e.g. D. Levy, S. Lorand) no longer regard the years between six and puberty as libidinally inactive; indeed, even in the children of Western cultures[4] there is a good deal of curiosity and exploration. What is more characteristic of the period, however, is the progressive channelization of the child's interests and activities into educational and social pursuits outide the immediate family. During this process the child partially transfers his libidinal relationships—dependent, aggressive or erotic—from his parents and siblings to various substitutes or *surrogates*: governesses, teachers, playmates, and others. Concurrently, the child may seek security in extrafamilial groups: his school, the neighborhood gang, his Boy Scout troop, or other associations which may mold the social patterns of the adult. This has long been recognized by religious bodies and thoroughly exploited by dictatorial regimes from Sparta to modern times.

*Puberty and Adolescence.* These, too, are periods of intensified adaptational stresses, when dependent, exploratory, erotic and other urges clash among themselves and add to the conflict between reawakened longings for the peace and security of childhood as opposed to tempting but anxiety-ridden drives to self-expression, emancipation, and freedom. Concurrently, the adolescent is faced with many problems: renewed friction with parental or school discipline, the multiple demands of scholastic, athletic, or sexual competitions with their attendant frustrations, the growing necessity of choosing a career, and other stresses that may appear portentous (Chapter 14). Adolescence, then, is characterized by many emotional hypersensitivities, deep concerns about personal appearance, accomplishments and revulsions, exaggerated self-assertiveness or regressive timidity, and a tendency to escapist fantasies.

It is at this time, too, that defects in earlier training become especially manifest: the unwanted or excessively punished child cringes before a world presumed to be forever inimical; adolescents who have been overprotected or overindulged by irresponsible parents are enraged because they can no longer fulfill burgeoning demands; those who had been covertly encouraged to act out their parents' own repressed wishes for unrestrained sex or vicarious aggression (*parental-superego lacunae*) now find that delinquent conduct is punished by others. Under effective guidance such youngsters may relearn and adapt; alternatively, they may retreat into puerile cynicism, disruptive attempts at defiant emancipation from social codes (Chapter 15, Case 7), or a breakdown into neurotic or psychotic patterns. Early adolescence may be the most difficult, and often the most poignantly unhappy time of life and is a period that requires the clearest understanding and most skillful handling on the part of parents, teachers, and physicians.

Personality development does not, of course, stop at adolescence, and there are later crises of stress and evolution: e.g., marriage, parenthood, the haunting reappraisals of late middle age (Chapter 14), and the regressions of senility (Chapter 15, Case 15).

## The Structure of the Personality

*The Id*[5]. This is conceived to be a repository of the "instincts" or drives of the individual expressed, as outlined above, in narcissistic, oral, anal, and genital *libidinal tendencies*, which constitute the *primary processes*. These are below the limen of the direct awareness of the individual, hence they comprise a large portion of what Freud reified as *the Unconscious*. Opposed to the primal conations of the Id are the repressive forces of the Ego (v.i.), which prevent inadmissible aggressive or erotic impulses from erupting into the awareness of the individual, pervading his behavior and so endangering his personal and social adjustments. In dreams this unconscious *censorship* and monitoring is relaxed, so that the undisciplined, unrealistic, unintegrated wishes of the Id, though still clothed in Ego-imposed allegory and symbolism, appear in more easily recognizable forms. Atavistic sexual or aggressive primary processes are likewise discernible, though less easily so, in fantasies, in free associations, in the hostile or erotic inadvertencies of speech and action (the *psychopathology of everyday life*) and in neurotic and psychotic symptom formation (Chapter 15, Cases 11,12).

*The Ego.* This designates a twofold function of the personality. The conscious Ego utilizes the information imparted by the senses, subjects these data to the discerning and integrative processes of the intellect, and so evaluates the milieu in terms of available sources and means of gratification as opposed to possible dangers of frustration or injury. Another aspect of the Ego, largely unconscious, is "directed inward" to oppose the forces of the Id by the use of various specific *secondary processes* or *defense mechanisms*.

## Defenses of the Ego

As elaborated by Freud's daughter Anna, these range from adaptive (numbers through 6 and 13 below) to neurotic (through 12) to psychotic (13 through 17). In essence, they are:

1. *Suppression*: the willful exclusion of dangerous antisocial motivations and affects from action.
2. *Denial*: the conscious refusal to accept unwelcome reality; e.g., internally, one's own conations, or externally, the news of the death of a loved person or the success of a hated one.
3. *Repression*: the *unconscious* inhibition of unacceptable impulses or affects so that, although they remain operative, they are not directly sensed or expressed.
4. *Displacement*: the transfer of meaning and value from one object, situation, or function to another; e.g., a girl may express postcoital concern over her "soiled genitals" by obsessive-compulsive oral hygiene.
5. *Undoing*: symbolic mitigation of a guilt; e.g., erecting a monument to a previously persecuted martyr.
6. *Substitution*: deviation of object-cathexes, either symbolic (e.g., devotion to pets in a woman deprived of children) or diverted (e.g., homosexuality due to heterosexual anxieties).
7. *Sublimation*: the channelization of repressed impulses into socially approved conduct; e.g., voyeurism into artistic body photography.
8. *Reaction formation*: rage against a frustrating loved one; e.g., heterosexual promiscuity in a repressed or disappointed homosexual.

9. *Phobia-formation*: dread of an object or situation symbolic of threat or conflict; e.g., fear of heights (*acrophobia*) in a patient who associates this with forbidden phallic eminence.

10. *Obsessive-compulsive reactions*: thoughts and/or acts that deny or conceal repressed memories or impulses; e.g., Lady Macbeth's incessant preoccupation with washing her hands to dispel the traces of homicide.

11. *Psychosomatic symptom formation*: expression of unconscious attitudes and conficts in musculoskeletal or internal visceral (organ neurotic) dysfunctions: e.g., chronic high blood pressure or joint pains in a patient who lives in a state of repressed anxiety or rage.

12. *Conversion reactions*: focalized sensorimotor (hysterical) dysfunctions; e.g., the onset of anesthesia and paralysis of the right arm in a man nearly overcome by an impulse to kill.

13. *Fantasy formation*: a recourse to wishful thoughts and imagery which may range from normal daydreams to the sensory misinterpretations (*illusions*), vivid imaginations, (*hallucinations*) and irrational convictions (*delusions*) of the psychotic.

14. *Projection*: the attribution of one's own motivations, ideas, and actions to others, as in feelings of being hated and persecuted (*paranoia*) in a person who wishes to justify his hostile intent toward others; if sufficiently generalized, this also leads to a compensatory *grandiosity*.

15. *Distortions of affect*: These comprise the emotional excesses of *euphoria* or *melancholy* in *manic-depressive reactions* versus the blunting or inappropriateness of affects in schizophrenia.

16. *Regression*: the resumption of modes of behavior that had been more satisfactory in earlier periods of life: e.g., the recurrence of infantile postures in *catatonia* or childlike conduct in *hebephrenia*.

In effect, the Ego is the interpretive, adaptive, and executive "part" of the personality, driven by the Id and conforming to the demands of the Superego as described below.

**The Superego.**[5]  In psychoanalytic parlance, the Superego denotes "a psychic apparatus" (constituting, with the Ego, a *secondary process*) that directs the primal strivings of the Id, as modified by the Ego, into behavior that further conforms to the double standards of the *conscience* and of the *Ego-Ideal*, differentiated as follows:

*The Conscience.*  In this capacity, the Superego is the repository of internalized prohibitions derived from the frustraneous, conflictful, and traumatizing experiences of childhood, and thereby consists of multiple pervasive "don'ts" which can be paraphrased variously as "thou shalt not preempt and incorporate aggressively," "thou shalt not soil and attack," "thou shalt not desire incest," and so on. In the early training of the child, these prohibitions acquire cogency from two main sources: fear of physical punishment from parents or parent-surrogates, or, far more serious to the helpless child, dread of loss of love should such parent-figures be displeased or injured by its actions.

Abnegations of dangerous and forbidden modes of behavior come to be regarded as a matter of self-preservation and of ultimate hedonic gain, and thereby become fixed in the adaptive patterns of the child. These self-imposed *inhibitions*, if later threatened by temptations or transgressed even in fantasy, or if flouted in action, occasion generalized apprehensions (*anxieties*) of varying intensity. Thus, the "conscience" derives its regulative powers from covert but persistent fears of punishment or deprivation—the ultimate source of all "guilt." Classical analytic theory holds that by the age of six the child has already run the gamut of narcissistic, incorporative, aggressive and erotic urges and their limens of retributions; hence his conscience is patterned relatively early in life and subsequent modifications become progressively more difficult.

*Cultural Influences.*  Karen Horney, Harry Sullivan, Abram Kardiner, Eric Fromm, and others have pointed out that, since the conscience is formed largely in accordance with parental, environmental and educational norms, the behavioral standards of adult individuals will vary widely from culture to culture.[6] A child raised along harsh authoritarian principles would be praised and rewarded even during his early formative years for behavior patterns that might be regarded elsewhere as ruthless, aggressive, and cruel, whereas he would be punished only for "transgressions against the family name" (or gang, party, church, state, etc.). Such a child grown to adulthood might feel "guilty" over ideologic disloyalty or military cowardice, but he would see no "wrong" in lying, stealing, or even murdering (v. the Hashishim) for the supposed good of his group. Fortunately, most children raised in democratic traditions adopt and live by humanitarian principles; however, a child strongly inculcated with antisocial attitudes by the precept and example of his parents might react to subsequent legal punishment by becoming more wary, but with little *internal* conflict or reorientation of values and objectives. Currently, an adult who sincerely insists on his good intentions but exhibits unconsciously determined compulsive, repetitive, and largely symbolic failures in social adaptation is termed a *sociopathic personality*; one who more deliberately plans preemptive and destructive antisocial acts is considered a criminal (Chapter 15, Case 7); finally, if the antisocial behavior became manifestly bizarre, dereistic, and delusional, his *criminal psychopathy* is treated with varying mixtures of psychologizing revenge.[7]

*The "Ego-Ideal".* This function of the Superego parallels and supplements the conscience, but controls behavior less by fear of consequences than by directing it toward accepted goals and standards. During the course of his social development the child derives such standards from various persons important in his environment whom he thereafter strives to emulate, not for idealistic reasons, but in a wishful attempt to attain the fancied advantages and prerogatives of the exemplar with whom he tries to *identify* (i.e., "introject"). For instance, a little girl playing with dolls is, in her own fancy, herself a "mother" with all her perquisites and privileges; just as in later life she will dress and gesture like the class belle or a popular actress so that she, too, may be a claimant to adoration and influence. Similarly, male youngsters cherish the trappings of glorified adulthood: cowboy, "Superman," or space explorer with toys that equate them with their powerful, envied (and feared) elders. More specific identifications with the traits of parents, teachers, or group leaders, or, later, artists, conquerors, or, for that matter, rebels or criminals may permanently mold the Ego-Ideal and so direct behavior into social or antisocial, successful or unsuccessful, and thereby "normal" or "neurotic" channels.

## TECHNIQUES OF PSYCHOANALYTIC THERAPY

Freud himself remained versatile in applying his developing theoretical concepts clinically, and, except for ethical standards, he set no rules for others as to the frequency, timing, or multiplicity of analytic hours. As one example, after a single session with Maestro Bruno Walter, Freud simply advised him to "disregard his neurosis" (a painful right arm) and return to conducting the Berlin Symphony Orchestra; as to other informalities, Freud treated some analysands while strolling with them through the Vienna woods. However, many of his disciples, first in England and then in the United States, began to require that every patient attend four or five 50-minute sessions per week for many years, lie on a couch facing away from the analyst, verbalize all current thoughts, recount dreams and fantasies, express all "emotions" (*v. catharsis* and *abreaction*), and discuss all attitudes toward the analyst. The latter, maintaining an ostensibly aloof objectivity, "interprets" all of these productions in terms of the patient's *unconscious*, his *ego defensive mechanisms*, his internalized *superego* prohibitions and aspirations, and his *transference relations*.[8] "*Insights*" so derived into the *perseveration* (persistent influence) of preoedipal "introjects" of persons significant in the patient's life are intended to remove his neurotic *fixations* on them, encourage new material and interpersonal interests (*object-cathexes*), relieve his inhibitions, and thus permit his adult intellect to redirect his libido into more "mature" (i.e., more realistic, creative, socially adaptive, and ultimately satisfactory) activities. As Freud put it: "Where Id was, there shall Ego be"—although some analysands reverse this to "where Ego was, there Id shall be."

Most psychoanalysts profess to limit their clientele to patients with anxiety states, phobic-obsessive-compulsive complaints, and the milder character neuroses; others accept sociopathic personalities with rebellious, irresponsible, self-frustrating patterns of conduct, recurrent *depressions* and even so-called *"borderline"* or *"schizoid"* personalities—quasi-psychotic individuals with only a veneer of adaptation to physical and cultural realities.

After 80 years of experience with "classical" psychoanalysis, the current consensus is that this prolonged, difficult, ritualized, and expensive mode of therapy may be instructive for professional students of the field and applicable to some carefully selected patients, but that shorter, more direct, and more versatile forms of dyadic influence are equally or more effective in most cases (Chapters 7 to 15).

## MODIFIED ANALYTIC TECHNIQUES

Those still professedly within the analytic framework (utilizing couch, free associations, dream interpretations, etc.) stress the following special aspects or objectives.

**Karen Horney.** Analysis is concentrated on the *social attitudes* of the patient (turning *toward, away from,* or *against* others) for the purpose of reestablishing individual responsibility and cultural participation. Horney eventually advocated explicit instructions as to social and moral duties.

**Franz Alexander.** This progressive leader in the field employed flexible schedules of interviews, daily diaries, written records of dream series, observation and interpretation of psychosomatic correlations, frank confrontations of the patient with the analyst's appraisals of his behavior to produce *reorientative emotional experiences* and a gradual diminution or a staggered suspension (*fractional analysis*) rather than a sudden termination of therapy.[9]

**Analyses of the Self.** Analysts of this school seek to elicit the unresolved residues of infantile self-love and the "introjection" of the all-powerful parent versus the rejections and frustrations of separation and "individuation" (Margaret Mahler).

Herewith a passage typical of speculative Self-school literature.[10]

> "The development of the ego and the striving for object relationship initially occur entirely between the infant and the mother.
>
> The important early people in the infant's world replace the superego.
>
> The baby grows and develops through a series of stages, beginning with a stage of hallucinatory fusion with the mother (the schizoid position). As the baby moves to some beginning separations, it enters a stage of oscillations between good and bad views of the environment (the paranoid position). Usually the baby emerges from this stage at between 6 and 12 months of age, depending in part on the mother's capacity to tolerate being seen by her baby as a witch and/or a saint. As the baby begins to accept that the mother is both good and bad simultaneously—and so in fact is he—he enters into a time of melancholic acceptance of this compromise (the depressive position).
>
> If all goes well, the baby develops the capacity for concern, the ability to love and hate simultaneously, and, incidentally, the capacity for feeling guilt."—Alonso and Rutan, 1984.

## DEVIATIONIST SCHOOLS

These were usually founded by colleagues of Freud who took exception to some of his basic tenets and techniques. The most prominent survivors are:

**The individual psychology of Alfred Adler,** which concentrates on correcting the *life style* of the patient by counteracting excessive feelings of inferiority and their exaggerated and impractical overcompensations or *masculine protests*. Therapy is supportive, reeducative, and directive.

**The analytic psychology of Carl Jung** is, by contrast, preoccupied with questionable dichotomies and typologies (logic vs. feeling: sensation vs. intuition: extravert vs. introvert), and a somewhat mystic search for a racial unconscious retained in an inaccessible anima (female) or animus (male) central to one's inner being. Therapy, which consists in part of philosophic discussions and shared intuitions about atavistic identifications, is often authoritative or nebulous.

**The approach of Otto Rank** was based on what he considered man's primary anxiety: the birth trauma consequent on the expulsion of the neonate from the nirvana of the mother's womb into an inimical external universe. Rank's depth analysis was charged with providing surrogate or material substitutes for the lost securities of the embryo and was for a time predictably popular with social workers; however, the Rankian and Jungian schools now have relatively few adherents in this country or elsewhere (A. Schmitt).

**Harry Stack Sullivan.** Practitioners of this subschool (R. Crowley, G. Chrzanowsky) define psychiatry as "the study of interpersonal (rather than "intrapsychic") relationships" and undertake a revision of the patient's actual normal or deviant (parataxic) dealings with his family, friends, and associates, as observed in his social as well as transference transactions. In hospital treatment, a "split transference" may be employed by assigning the conflicting duties of permissive analyst and corrective disciplinarian to separate therapists.

There are many other deviants from Freudian psychoanalysis. The disciples of Melanie Klein believe that analysis must reach down to the *primal depressions* and *paranoid states* of the first 6 weeks of life; the radical French cult of Jacques Lacan holds sessions that vary from 10 minutes to all day, with hostile harangues when indicated. Angel Garma of the Argentine School personalizes the concepts of "bad introjects" to the extent of attributing gastric ulcers to oral attacks on the mucosa by a vengeful mother; and the scattered acolytes of the late Willhelm Reich still accept the notion that the universe is permeated by a form of ethereal libido which can be collected in patented *orgone boxes* for the restoration of sexual potency (D. Elkind).

As I have indicated elsewhere, such protean "insight therapies" may be defined dynamically as temporary or permanent states comparable to a *folie à deux* in which patients and analysts share the same illusions—sometimes as counterproductive as salutory. Fortunately, therapeutic results depend far less on the theories held than on the influences of an empathetic analyst, whatever his persuasion, in helping his patient achieve a better adapted, more creative, and thereby happier life, by utilizing any combination of the therapeutic modalities developed in this volume.

## Notes

1.  H. Harlow has shown that baby monkeys cling to furry inanimate "mothers" with greater avidity than they seek food; so also, Bowlby (1959) believes that maternal bodily contact is the single most important source of security in infancy and of amity in later life. The "Cornelian Corner" (named for Cornelia, the Roman noblewoman who proclaimed "my only jewels are my children") is a national organization dedicated to promoting early bodily intimacies between mother and child.

2.  For a detailed psychoanalysis of a patient with anorexia nervosa *v.* Masserman, 1946, Appendix I.

3.  Sandor Ferenczi fancifully correlated this with the Ice Ages in racial development.

4.  B. Malinowsky, M. Mead, G. Bateson and other anthropologists have observed no "latency period" whatever in sexually uninhibited cultures.

5.  The Id-Superego-Ego trilogy is interestingly reminiscent of the battles of Seth, Ahreman, Loki, Satan, and other subversive devils in various theologies (the Id) who contend with im-

perious Ra, Ahura Mazda, Brahma, or Yaweh (the Superego) for the control of human behavior as mediated by demigods such as Engedu, Mithra Osiris, or Moses (the Ego).

6. Margaret Mead reported that in some cultures (as among the Arapesh), late weaning and the encouragement of almost every form of oral satisfaction in children may establish feelings of infantile security which persist into adult life, and so contribute to the formation of a stable, content, and relatively noncompetitive society. However, A. Gesell's dictum is here pertinent: "It is very apparent that the human infant assimilates the cultural milieu only by gradual degrees; that he has vast immunities to acculturation; that his nervous system sets metes and bounds to what the societal group would do for him; indeed, determines what is done. The culture is adapted to him, primarily; he adapts when he is ready."

7. The very word "mores" is the plural of the Latin *mos* (custom) meaning a social pattern devoid of implications of morality. J. Peters (1933) put it trenchantly: "There is perhaps not a single vice in the code of our own society that some other group has not considered a virtue—murder, theft, dishonesty, torture, suicide, adultery and the rest."

8. Much as a child will project his dependence, resentments, or other attitudes toward parents and siblings later onto school peers, teachers, or others, a patient may "transfer" onto his therapist the reliance, envy, suspicion, or ambivalent love and hostility toward others previously important in his life, rendering the detection of such *neurotic transferences* helpful in clarifying interpersonal relationships outside the analysis. However, some analysts insist that an erotic, aggressive, or otherwise artificial *transference neurosis* should be deliberately engendered in order to be resolved—a practice reminiscent of the "laudable pus" that medieval surgeons insisted must occur as necessary for good surgery.

9. For an account of my personal analyses by Dr. Alexander, see Masserman, *A Psychiatric Odyssey*, 1970.

10. Self-analysts do not trouble to explain how the as yet unmyelinated cerebrum of a neonate can develop "introjects" that will dominate the rest of its life (until presumably, cor-

rected by a Self-analyst)—let alone how such character patterns can be labelled empirically as "schizoid", "depressive" or "paranoid". Otto Kernberg and Heinz Kohut present different views as to how and when such "libidinally good" (narcissistically augmenting) or "bad" (depreciative or conflictful) introjects occur, with their concomitant effects on "splitting the Ego" and thus creating a "borderline personality"; however, their somewhat turgid prose and involuted polemics have little or no demonstrable relevance to effective therapy.

Chapter 9

# DIVERSE DYADIC THERAPIES[1]

These combine so great a variety of modalities as to render meaningless group distinctions among "physical" *vs* "psychologic," "directive" vs. "persuasive," "deep" vs. "superficial," or even rational vs. mystical; for ease of reference, they are therefore listed merely in alphabetical order. Cultist procedures, usually under the name of their originator or promoter, are entered briefly; those more widely practiced receive fuller discussions as to their physical, interpersonal, or metapsychologic dynamics.

**Alexander Technique** (F.M.M. Alexander) employs "cosmically systematized" bodily caresses and massages designed to elicit memories, thoughts, and desires that "enhance creative living."

**Attention Antenna Therapy** (M. J. Meldman) relies on an "orienting antenna" attached to a patient's eyeglasses to receive and recall the therapist's messages as a diversion from fears of crowds or open spaces.

**Autogenic Training** (J. H. Schultz) prescribes regulated breathing, muscular exercises and ritualized "auto-suggestions" designed to induce "mind-body harmony."

**Autosuggestion** (E. Coué) *sine* exercises, employs some lilting self-administered formula (i.e., "every day in every way I am getting better and better") whenever required as a psychologic *aperitif.*

**Bibliographic Therapy.** Religious, technical, fictional, or poetic sources may range from the Bible, through Boccaccio and Shakespeare to *Zen and the Art of Archery.* Adherents of *est* (see Chapter 11) are directed to peruse Werner Erhard; psychoanalytic trainees must study most of Freud's writings, and members of Recovery, Inc. must quote Abraham Low's *Mental Health through Will Power* at every meeting. Directed readings may help in the acquisition of knowledge, inculcate social graces, elicit talents and develop adaptive and creative conduct through identification with real or fictional characters. Regrettably, poorly selected literature (as in some self-help groups,) may be counterproductive in all of these respects.

**Bioenergetics** (A. Lowen, derived from W. Reich's "orgoneology"). Prescribed breathing and massage (with the patient preferably nude); pelvic thrusts and other muscular rituals "break through emotional tensions" and "body armor" to "release erotic and aggressive energies," in either dyadic or group sessions.

**Biofeedback** (M. Hamm). Subjects observe mechanical or electronic indicators of their alpha brain waves (electroencephalograms), muscular tensions (myograms), heart rate (electrocardiograms), blood pressure (Doppler flowmeters), or other somatic functions, and then endeavor consciously to control them by responding to self-administered signals. This "somatic condioning" may be combined with transcendental meditation (B. Glueck), muscular relaxation (E. Jacobson), "auto-hypnosis" (T.X. Barber), or other modalities.

**Child Therapies.** These comprise a panoply of techniques, many derived from adult procedures as suited to children of various ages. Examples are art (finger-painting, M. Naumberg), costume therapy (I. Marcus), dance, the George Junior Republic "for training in democracy" (R.E. Pittenger), music or mutual story-telling (R.A. Gardner), puppetry and play techniques (A. Freud, R.E. Hartley, & R.M. Goldenson), and pet therapy (S.A. Corson).

**Client-centered Therapy** (Carl Rogers; I.H. Paul). The verbalizations of "clients" are noncommitally mirrored in question form to foster reciprocal "self-actualization." The former designation of "nondirective therapy" was abandoned as too easily confused with "noncorrective."

**Clothing Therapy** (Cho & Grover). Self-expression through raiment.

**Computer Feedback** (K. Colby) consists of having a programmed computer respond with noncommital comments (e.g.: "yes? . . ." "what do you think?" . . . "please go on") to a patient's verbal or typed input, thereby evoking elaboration of, and presumably alleviating, anxieties, inhibitions, phobias, compulsions, or other aberrations without need for physician or cleric. Such programmed feedback may include recommendations for nonprescription drug therapy (J. Maxmen).

**Counting Therapy** (George Saslow) directs subjects to keep accurate tab of the number of times per hour or day they experience thoughts or actions that are to be corrected by behavior techniques (Chapter 10).

**Dianetics** (L. Ron Hubbard). An "auditor," who has himself been properly "audited" and commissioned by the "Church of Scientology," listens to the semidirected expressions of a recumbent subject until the latter's "engrams" of ostensibly fateful life experiences, including perinatal or even embryonic ones, are "ventilated" and, by dramatic abreaction, "cleared" of their "subconsciously" disturbing effects (v. Primal Scream).

**Do In** (J. Hart). The therapist, through exhortations and various forms of massage, transfers to the subject *ki*, a form of energy that allegedly maximizes vitality and potency.

**Existential Therapies.** L. Binswanger advocates "unprejudiced and non-judgmental interpersonal observations" (as though these are possible) as essential "to therapeutic empathy." Applied clinically, existential modalities entail a somewhat esoteric melange of perceptions of one's "cosmic autonomy" through concentrating on one's *dasein* ("I am there") or "vital being" (Camus). Sociocultural alienations are countered by encouraging I-Thou acceptances (the intimate *begegnungen* of M. Buber) and death itself by a Beethovian defiance (S. Kierkegaard; J.P. Sartre) (Chapter 14).

**Humor Therapy** (E. Rosenheim) employs the amieliorative effects of cogently witty observations and interpretations without resorting to the "tickle therapy" of A. Selma.

**Interactional Therapy** (Don Jackson) permits unusual techniques, such as directing a masculine-orienting woman to smoke the therapist's pipe to cure her warts (they disappeared), or using hypnosis to transfer another subject's facial tic to her shoe-encased big toe so that "it didn't annoy others."

**Living Love** teaches adherents (as did Omar Khayyam) that since the past is unchangeable and the future ephemeral, wisdom dictates enjoying the present to the fullest, while "playing life's game intensively . . . win or lose."

**Mentor Therapy** (Robert Burton) advocates that the therapist, after resolving the patient's unconscious conflicts, should continue to act as an examplar, advisor and guide indefinitely.

**Metapsychiatry** (J. Eisenbud; cf. S. Freud's "the Uncanny," and C. Jung's "Universal Unconscious,") utilizes "*psi* phenomena" and intuitive, premonitory, clairvoyant, dream, telepathic, and other forms of extrasensory communication for esoteric therapeutic purposes. (For a phenomenologic and methologic critique, see D. Rawcliffe).

**Mind Control** ("Yoga is its mother, and hypnosis its father" —Jose Silva). Week-end seminars consist of exercises such as printing a "difficult question of living" on a black-framed mirror, changing the frame to white and thereby enlightening and abolishing the problem. Diseases can be similarly diagnosed and cured by telepathy through "levels of consciousness" empathetic with inanimate as well as animate objects.

**Morita Therapy,** as first practiced by Prof. Shama Morita in Japan, consisted of an initial period of enforced bed rest, meditative introspections recorded in a diary, and a strictly prescribed, graduated and supervised work regimen. After several weeks, the patient was discharged with authoritative instructions that, if his duties were properly performed, doubts, inhibitions, and physical symptoms would either diminish or must be stoically borne. After importation to the West (D. Reynolds) there have been endless variations toward a more sympathetic and individualized approach in both in-patient and out-patient therapy.

**Nonagenic Therapy** (M. Tyndell). Forensic action by the therapist protects against false arrests, imprisonment for alcoholism, and other juristically induced stresses.

**Occupational Therapy** (J. Weinroth; L. Linn) cultivates manual skills, and pride of accomplishment in individual or joint endeavors to restore lost self-confidence in an encouraging and rewarding milieu of work, but may be misused to serve a repressive social system.

**Paradoxical Therapy** (Allen Fay) sarcastically exaggerates the patient's complaints; *Tantric Therapy* mirrors behavioral absurdities to reveal and correct their aberrations.

**Persuasion** (W. Dubois; V. Dejerine). The therapist employs logical dialectics in appeals to the patient's self-interest to change his conduct for the better. (In various forms from gentle to semicoersive, persuasion is an element in nearly every form of therapy).

**Poetry Therapy** (J. Leedy; A. Lerner; J. Masserman) utilizes the metaphoric subtleties of poetic language to illumine hidden truths, inspire verbal creativity, and promote interpersonal communication.

**Posture Therapy** (Moshe Feldenkreis, derived from the "body-dynamics" of G. Enelow) teaches scores of poses and exercises designed to reestablish self-confidence by "integrating the mind with the body."

**Psychoimagination** (J. Shorr) "actualizes" the patient's imagery in quasi-realistic situations so that he can experience and resolve his "intrapsychic anxieties and conflicts" by mobilizing his untapped "ego strengths" for "corrective conduct." Psychocybernetics (M. Maltz) is a more pretentious and directive predecessor.

**Puppet Therapy** (P. Kors) employs movable dolls manipulated by patients to represent figures in life or fantasy. Conflicts and their resolution can thus be dramatized and resolved in dyadic or group settings.

**Rational-Emotive Therapy** (A. Ellis) corrects the patient's "misleading concepts." As summarized by J. Marmor, these are "(a) that it is necessary to be loved and approved by everyone; (b) that one must be thoroughly competent, adequate, and achieving in all respects in order to consider oneself worthwhile; (c) that human unhappiness is caused by external circumstances over which one has no control; (d) that it is easier to avoid life's difficulties than to face them; (e) that one needs to be dependent on others and have someone stronger than oneself on whom to rely; and (f) that there is a correct, precise, and perfect solution to all human problems and that it is catastrophic not to have found it." Ellis also advocates considerable sexual freedom for both patient and therapist.

**Rebirthing** (R. Harper) symbolically corrects the trauma of birth (O. Rank) by submerging the subject in a tub of water while he breathes through a snorkel reciprocally with the therapist. This is followed by a dramatic "delivery," accompanied by reassurances by the therapist and a celebrant group that the neonate's primal fears will be forever dispelled in his new life as a born-again adult.

**Redecision Therapy** (M.M. & R.L. Goulden) mixes Gestalt, transactional, imagery, and other modalities intended to induce a patient "to alter his life plans."

**Relaxation Exercises** (E. Jacobson) combined bodily "repose" with "mind training" in 1891, and others have followed with various methods for relaxing "muscle tensions" to cure various disorders ranging from onychocryptosis[2] to migraine.

**Rest Cures** (Weir Mitchell) combined diets, massage, electrostimulation and enforced isolation with avuncular lectures as a panacea for overintensive life styles. A modern version is proposed by D.V. Treffert (see below).

**Rolfing** (Ida Rolf) "aligns the body . . . [with the sun's rays] . . . and with the earth's gravity fields" and employs vigorous and often painful pummeling and massage to "release locked energy," which can then be channeled by explicit instructions as to proper conduct. The method seems to combine a maternal spanking with solicitous or hortatory parental guidance.

**Social Skill Therapy** (L.S. Zegans; A. Bellak) counters interpersonal inhibitions, phobias, or compulsions by the verbal and nonverbal training of patients in the amenities of interpersonal actions, trusting that adaptive inner reorientations will follow.

**Supportive Therapy** (L.R. Wolberg) utilizes guidance, "tension control and release", environmental manipulation, externalization of interests, and reassurances. Wolberg states that, contrary to psychoanalytic dogma, "mere symptom relief," instead of "inhibiting progress" may instead lead to salutory and permanent personality change.

**T'ai Chi** comprises a routine of postural exercises imported from China that epitomize neuromuscularly the Yin/Yang principles of interacting tension and relaxation, thereby providing mental concentration and competence "to cope with and integrate cosmic contradictions." (Wu Chi)

**Telepsychiatry.** Telephones (D. Lester) or closed-circuit tele vision (C. Wittson, T.Dwyer) permit two-way communication between a therapist and a distant patient at home, at an airport, the scene of an accident, or elsewhere.

**Transcendental Meditation** (Maharishi Mahesh Yogi; P. Carrington; for relationships to Zazen, see Tomio Hirai). An authorized practitioner provides a confidentially prescribed "mantra" for the subject to repeat during two daily 20-minute periods of silent, restful contemplation designed to restore a sense of wholeness and "cosmic relatedness." The Maharishi teaches that when 5 percent of the world's population practice TM, disease, crime, and war will disappear and the weather will also improve. For those who wish greater transcendence, the Maharishi International University offers doctorate degrees in the Science of Creative Intelligence, and an advance course at only $375 per week promises the ability to levitate, fly, and dematerialize. Parenthetically, what may also be called *transcendental medication* (T. Leary) employs psychedelic drugs to enhance vividness of imagery and disinhibitions of conduct.

**Vegetotherapy** (W. Reich) directs subjects to sit in metallic closets which accumulate cosmically ubiquitous "orgone energy" that reactivates the "vegetative nervous system" and thereby cures afflictions ranging from impotence to cancer. Despite federal restrictions, Reichian devices are still operating in many parts of the country, as are relics of the era of animal magnetism, magic belts, protective copper necklaces, and other thaumaturgic amulets.

**Verbal and Operant Directives.** H. Rheder assured three severely ill patients that at a precise moment a famous faith healer in a distant city would alleviate their suffering. All three showed an immediate and lasting improvement at the specified time, although the absent healer had actually acted a day previously, when no effects had been observed.

On a more literally "operant" plane (Chapter 10) ligation of the mammary artery was for years thought to be an effective method for shunting blood to a failing heart—until Beecher and Ross demonstrated that a mere incision of the skin of the chest in anesthetized cardiac patients produced equally beneficient results.

**Yoga** (N. Vahia) *Zen* (Buddha Bahrdedarma) and similar cults employ master-votary discipline to teach Oriental tenets of abnegation, body repose, affective control, and evolving levels of "enlightenment" as an approach to the selfless peace of "perfect illumination," (*nirvana*) with or without cultist religious (e.g., Krishna Consciousness) connotations. Rami Yogi (Shri Swami Rama) teaches regulated postures and muscular exercises (*sarvangasana*) and ritualized breathing through alternate nostrils (*prana*) designed to distribute bodily energies (*chakras*) and elevate consciousness until a state of selflessness (*samadhi*) facilitates "pure, focused meditation." *Tantric Yoga* permits occasional escapes from austerity to satisfy physiologic and erotic needs so that serene detachment can return.

**Zootherapy** (S.A. Corson) utilizes animal pets (S. Wood) on the principle that when no one else seems to care, a parrot will ask for a cracker, a cat will cuddle and purr, and a dog will tender unequivocal loyalty and affection even to the mentally retarded, the schizophrenic, or the incapacitated aged.

Since all of these modalities, many at high fees, have received public support, they have manifestly offered their votaries physical, social, or metapsychologic (Ur) benefits; however, there are few valid follow-up studies as to their lasting effects. Proponents of behavior and group therapies, as described in the following chapters claim greater credibility in this respect.

## NOTES

1. For bibliographic references to Chapters 9, 10 and 11, cf Masserman, 1978.

2. See my pseudoanalytic derivation of the "psychosomatic formula for ingrown toenails" (Masserman, *The Practice of Dynamic Psychiatry*, 1955, pp. 474-476).

# Chapter 10

# BEHAVIOR THERAPIES

Based on the studies of animal behavior by Sechenov, Pavlov, Liddell, Skinner, N.E. Miller, and the author (Chapter 5),[1] various therapists, particularly clinical psychologists, began to apply concepts of "behavior conditioning" to their patients some 40 years ago. Agras has defined this approach as follows: "The [behavior therapists] . . . assume that problem behavior is maintained by its consequences. Thus, to change behavior it is necessary to change those consequences and to arrange an environment in which appropriate new behavior can be learned. [Behavior therapy removes] symptoms directly . . . in the life situation in which [they] occur [while substituting] desired behavior . . . in a specially designed program."

**Terminology.** *Eliciting stimuli* induce either *attractive* or *aversive* responses. Attractive stimuli (e.g., to food) can be enhanced by *secondary reinforcers* (e.g., a pleasant setting); aversive stimuli (e.g. nauseating substances) by deterrents (e.g., odors, censure). *Elicited responses* are then *generalized* through *relevant associations* (e.g. to books on gourmet cooking), or *confined* or *extinguished* by prolonged deprivation or social disdain. *Operant* *conditioning* occurs when a *manipulation* (e.g., a kiss) acts as *positive reinforcer*, whereas a *negative* one may be a slap[2] or conversely, the removal of an obstacle to desired behavior (B.F. Skinner). Birk et. al. exemplify combinations of various terms as follows:

"A *chain* (e.g., party going) usually begins with . . . a *discriminative stimulus* (e.g., a phone invitation) [and] an appropriate *response* (e.g., acceptance) followed by a *conditioned reinforcer* (e.g., 'Glad you can make it'). This is also the *discriminative stimulus* for the next *appropriate response* (e.g., washing, dressing) that in turn is followed by another *conditioned reinforcer* (e.g., leaving the house, catching a cab) which is also a *discriminative stimulus* for the next response (e.g., joining the party). . . . Such *chains* are maintained by the intermittent . . . occurrences of potent consequences (e.g., food, sex) [or terminated by frustration or tedium]."

### TECHNIQUES OF THERAPY

**Desensitization.** In this modality, bodily repose is first induced in accord with various suggestions by the therapist. Fears of objects, situations, or actions are then "reciprocally inhibited" by reassociating them with pleasant stimuli; provided by either the therapist or patient, or merely imagined. Thus, a subject afraid of heights may be induced to climb to the second floor of a building by fantasying, or being actually provided with a potential sex partner inviting him to climb gradually higher until he can gaze over the edge of a 20-story building with or without a promissory Circe. (Birk describes more explicit sexual modalities for impotence or frigidity). Similar methods of associating "positive" with previously "negative" stimuli have been reported to be successful for child terrors (Abramovitz), adult insomnia (Geer & Katkin), and exhibitionism (Birk). Soldiers suffering from combat neuroses were permitted to control the duration, noise level, and context of war films to the point of tolerance before being returned to military action (Chapter 15, Case 8). The author relieved a prominent executive of a career-threatening fear of flying by having him first fly in the author's small plane and then act as co-pilot—after which the patient not only trusted commercial transports but secured his own pilot's license.

**Behavior Economics.** Ayllon and Azrin instructed attendants in a psychiatric ward: first, to treat recalcitrant patients with "benign neglect" until they became more cooperative, and then to reward them appropriately with colored plastic "coins" exchangeable for home visits and other privileges. These combined "negative and positive reinforcements" produced favorable improvements in self-care, increased participation in educational or occupational retraining, and amelioration of withdrawn or irrational conduct.[3] Other settings require token systems more suitable to the milieu: in grammar school, a gold star for parental approval; in industry, a citation (sometimes in lieu of a raise); in military service, a good conduct stripe in anticipation of promotion. Freer environments involve more complexly symbolic compensations.

**Aversion Techniques.** These aim to diminish or eliminate "target behaviors" by pairing them with unpleasant stimuli; i.e., for alcoholism, an emetic coupled with the smell or taste of ethyl liquors (M. Voegtlin); or, for homosexuals, an electric shock simultaneous with the exhibition of the genitals of a same-sex partner. Results are uncertain: one may be that the alcoholic learns to shun emetics and the homosexual all electrical appliances.

**Deterrence.** In 1812 Dr. Benjamin Rush (v. Chapter 2) stated that "psychopathic behavior" was to be treated by purging, bloodletting, tranquilizing chairs to which patients were chained, "whipping when necessary," and other such measures. In current behavioral modalities, the symptom to be extinguished (e.g., head-banging in children; threats or tantrums in adults) meets with *symbolically* dissuasive stimuli; e.g., withdrawal of desired attention, including, when necessary, enforced seclusions (*times out*), followed by suitable rewards when better conduct supervenes. These procedures may modify specific "target traits," but they produce little generalization unless supplemented by consistent familial and social reinforcers (Liberman) (Chapter 15, Case 2).

**Assertiveness Training.** "[Excitatory social reflexes are substituted for inhibitory ones] in teaching overly meek, anxious, or apologetic persons to be firm in their convictions and effective, though not domineering or belligerent, in their interpersonal relationships" (J.M. Ferguson). Techniques include "modeling" by the therapist and audio or video feedbacks of role-playing in psychodramatic groups (R. Lomont)—presumably with appropriate cautions to adapt the newly acquired skills to social parameters. According to a 1979 survey, behavior therapists currently prefer assertiveness training, biofeedback and "rational emotive therapy" to other techniques (Wade & Hartmann).

**Flooding.** The subject is induced in rapidly graduated escalations to imagine a feared situation (e.g., standing at the edge of a precipice), or actually to experience it until his panic abates. In a variant termed *paradoxical intention*, a patient afraid of syncope is encouraged or commanded to faint—and finds he cannot. Similar procedures to establish controlled stoicism are termed *aragamama* in Japanese Morita therapy. Such procedures, including the physical prevention of obsessive-compulsive rituals, must be carefully selected and modulated with respect to the subject's tolerance and flexibility, else they may constitute seriously traumatic experiences with exacerbated phobic and aversive effects (Masserman, 1946).

**Contingency Contracts.** Mutually rewarding behaviors can be expedited by clear "contracts" among participants. Such arrangements may be emplicitly or explicitly applied to patient-therapist interactions and extended to familial, school, group industrial, and social conduct.

### Recent Critiques

"The trend away from the behavioristic paradigm has become all but a stampede, as the resurgence of cognitive psychology illustrates" (W.B. Weimer).

"[A therapeutic] relationship is a necessary, if not a sufficient, condition for meaningful improvement. This can never be explained by conditioning theories that focus [merely] on . . . acquisition, generalization, and extinction (de Voge & Beck). However, since most behavior therapists now acknowledge that genetic predispositions, and sociocultural experiences result in preconceptions, contingent motivations, symbolic values and current interpersonal relationships unique to each patient, most "behavior therapies," despite rear-guard protests such as those of J. Wolpe, converge in theory and practice with more comprehensive and dynamic modalities of treatment.

## NOTES

1. Masserman, *Behavior and Neuroses*, 1946.

2. However, it is important to differentiate what the subject regards as reward or punishment: a spanking may be a desired attention to a misbehaving child.

3. However, "Forgery of tokens is not unknown, or stealing, or 'borrowing' with coercion. . . Patients go into business and lend, charging interest, or sell items at a profit when the commissary is closed." (W.S. Agras) Because of such problems one of every four token programs in Veterans Administration Hospitals has been discontinued (Stegner & Peck).

*Chapter 11*

# GROUP AND METAPSYCHOLOGIC THERAPIES

These offer the following advantages:

> Group choices and participation in music, dance, plays, and other activities of constructive social value;
>
> A changing membership to accommodate diverse personalities;
>
> Generally lowered costs per patient;
>
> Salutary post-group contacts among members and with the therapist.

Reciprocally, therapists can observe, participate in, and influence a multitude of therapeutic interactions, and develop a versatility of techniques in orienting the group experience to social realities outside the office, clinic, or institution.

### GROUP ANALYTIC AND BEHAVIORAL TECHNIQUES

Among the scores of modalities, many offered by nonprofessionals, those of primary therapeutic interest are outlined below.

**Arica** (Oscar Tschazo) offers an "open door" to removing "disturbing desires" and restoring "infantile innocence" through mystic meditations, readings of Tarot cards, chants, dances, contemplation of *mantras*, and recitations of magical *yantras*.

**Art Therapy** (M. Naumberg, M. Horowitz) develops pictorial and esthetic skills and visually actualizes fantasies for interpretation in a receptive dyadic or group milieu. Motion pictures are made and exhibited for group reactions (C. Muller).

**Community Services.** These are based on the thesis that just as society is charged with the prevention as well as the treatment of communicable diseases, so also is it responsible for averting behavior disorders insofar as possible or treating them in their earliest stages. The following services are therefore provided.

*Counseling for students and teachers* in the school systems from kindergarden through college, with special attention to actual or potential scholastic failures, premature dropouts, teenage pregnancies, and the growing problems of drugs and delinquency.

*Consultation services* for police, welfare, and other federal, state, and municipal departments as to internal personnel policies and programs that affect social cohesion, security, and morale.

*Out-patient clinics and specialized suicide prevention centers* to which persons in desperate straits and suffering extreme despondency can appeal at any hour for interim aid and restoration of hope.

*Day hospitals* designed for the individual and group treatment of patients who would benefit by retained contact with their home and family.

*Night hospitals* which furnish evening and night-time therapy for patients while they are kept beneficially employed.

*Wards in general hospitals* where patients requiring full-time care can be admitted for short periods without the onus of legal proceedings.

*Community zone centers* as developed in Illinois (H. Visotsky) and New York (R. Campbell) in which all of these services are combined with research and teaching.

*Prolonged treatment hospitals* for more serious or chronic illnesses, some of which may require court commitment of the patient.

**Crisis Therapy** (D. Langsley) for rapid reorientations of behavior under skillfully directive familial, group, institutional, and social guidance. Hospital emergency rooms often offer a triage setting (D. Muller) for especially effective action.

**Dance Therapy** (Marian Chase) supplemented by music (see Music Therapy) fosters spontaneous self-expression or group relationships through synchronous bodily movements and contacts (R. Birdwhistell). Costumes (J. Marcus) may enhance a variety of roles and interactions.

**Environmental or Milieu Therapies** utilize half-way houses for rehabilitative care (G. Wayne). Full-time retreats for alcoholics, drug addicts or others in need of continuous periods of supervision employ medical care, individual counseling and occupation and other group modalities.

**Esalin** formerly provided surcease from customary stresses in weekend or longer periods in seaside or mountain resorts. Co-founder Richard Price, now called Swami Geel Govind, is also directing Esalin toward "instant enlightenment via the cult of Bhagwan Shree (Sir God) Rajneesh." In other "retreats" or "therapeutic communities," participants are promised relief from personal responsibilities through seemingly paradoxical but complementary policies: sexual and other permissiveness at the price of strict adherence to the dictates of charismatic leaders (v. Synanon). If the cult, as in the case of the more widely dispersed enclaves of the *Church of Scientology*, secures recognition as a religious body, it acquires financial and other immunity in its crusades against mental health professionals.

**EST** (Erhard Seminar Training, W. Erhard) employs weekends of physical confinement, bodily discomforts, challenging harangues, and a variety of marathon endurance tests to teach participants, at considerable cost, to "face their deficiencies and failures . . . generate new attitudes not from experience but from nothing," and so attain *it*—conceived as a form of quasicynical, quasi-existential self-sufficiency.[2]

**Exercise Therapy** (E. Smallwood) enhances body image and feelings of physical competence, either solipsistically (barbells, golf, T'ai chi), jogging (T. Kostrubala), or in military drill.

**Family Therapy.** By acting as an observer, recorder, moderator, interpreter, advocate, conciliator, or in other roles, the therapist (N. Ackerman; I. Alger,) elicits, clarifies, and improves familial and other interpersonal relationships. Genetic counseling (J. Rainer) can be extended to multiple couples (H.P. Laqueur) or "family-network" transactions (R.V. Speck). Crises may require particularly active intervention or family hospitalization (A. Gralnick) (Chapter 15, Cases 9,13).

**Geriatric Therapy** requires familial environments, transference dependencies, and treatment procedures that best accommodate the declining physical, psychologic, affective, and interpersonal capacities and mitigate the loneliness and alienation of the aged. (Chapter 15, Cases 14,15). Comfort for the dying may include medication for pain and anxiety, family support, and pastoral counseling.

**Gestalt Therapy** (F. Perls, E. Marcus, C. Hatcher). By enforcing minute self-observation of "bodily needs" and by pooling group accounts of dreams, fantasies, and desires, Gestalt techniques effect "closures" among repressed, unsatisfied, or disparate categories of motivations, affects, and experiences "between the Self and others." The therapist asks "How?" but considers the analytic Why? a "trap." Gestalt therapy aims for a "holistic reunion of personality, environment, and society in the here and now [not] then and there... Integration and responsibility are key objectives." Associated techniques employ existential (H. Kelman) and psychoanalytic (W. Kohler) concepts. Psychodramatic, and "expressive techniques" include hugging, kissing, and more intense erotic activities.

**Integrated Therapies** (F.K. Knobloch & J. Knobloch). A clinic, a residential community, and a day center are flexibly utilized in "seven steps": (1) introductory interviews that avoid "evasive cliches" and stress explicit goals in therapy; (2) preliminary orientations in groups of 18 to 24 new, treated, and former patients; (3) 4 to 6 weeks of work and recreation in a regulated rural community; (4) rapprochement contacts with "significant persons"; (5) group follow-up for extramural rehabilitation; (6) renewed individual or family therapy as indicated, leading to (7) membership in clubs of expatients and friends. (Compare with the 7 R's of dynamic therapy outlined in Chapter 3).

**Marathon Therapy** (T. Casriel). Batteries of therapists conduct hours or days of unremitting "togetherness" for verbal and physical interactions until "interpersonal alienations" are shattered in mutual exhaustion.

**Military Therapy** (A. Glass) adds to other forms of treatment the advantages of authoritative discipline, common interests or dangers, and consequent group *esprit*.

**Music Therapy** (E.T. Gaston; J. Masserman) employs the rhythm, melody, harmony, and counterpoint plus the delight of musical performance to supplement other physical, dyadic, and group modalities.

**Penal Therapy** deals with the often conflicting roles of the therapist variously conceived as friend and counsellor versus warden or spy (S. Halleck).

**Self-Help Groups** are formed to aid specifically troubled persons to resolve individual, familial, or social difficulties in an atmosphere of confidentiality, mutual understanding, and conjoint effort, with or without professional guidance. Typical are Addicts Anonymous, Alcoholics Anonymous (which claims to aid half its applicants), Debtors Anonymous, Encounter (Sensitivity or T) Groups, Gamblers Anon., Human Potential Meetings, Integrity Sessions, Mattachine (homosexual) Societies, Neurotics Anonymous, Overeaters Anonymous, Parents of Gays, Parents of Retarded (or otherwise handicapped) Children, Parents Without Partners, Prostitutes Anonymous, and Widows Anonymous, all apparently striving symbolically for Recovery, Inc. (A. Low). As indicated by their names, most of these groups have a unitary, peer-oriented, and quasi-missionary purpose to rescue members from isolation, alienation, and despair and to support them while acquiring an improved outlook and style of life. Meetings generally follow a special routine, sometimes with covert religious or moralistic overtones. Sessions may or may not be open to the public.

When members fit in, they are often helped; however, recidivists and dropouts may react with increased feelings of failure and rejection. Regrettably, also, some groups use as texts the current avalanche of "self-help" books such as *The Joy of Sex*, *Looking Out For No. 1* (D. Biggs, M. Shepard, et al.) that, in effect, counsel narrowly solipsistic conduct, ultimately with socially adverse results.

**Synanon** (C. Diderich) is representative of a number of "retreats," "communes," "extended families" (now interconnected by a fleet of planes and private airports) or other such sometimes militant congregates that offer well-paying participants a temporary escape from life's extramural stresses (E. Markoff).

**Transactional Therapies.** These are usually associated with the "personality structure" and "game" concepts of Eric Berne, which may be summarized as follows:
Every person may assume an *extero-*, *neo-*, or *arche-psychic* "ego state," roughly corresponding, in analytic terminology, to superego, ego, and id (Chapter 8). Accordingly, he may conduct

himself as a *Parent* (nurturing, authoritative, or punitive), as an *Adult* (realistic, forethoughtful, adaptational), or as a *Child* (subservient, free, or reckless). Two persons, when transactionally "hooked," can thereby interact variously in *Parent↔Child, Adult↔Adult,* or *Child↔Adult* vectors, each with almost an infinity of derived nuances at various psychological or social "open" or "locked" levels. The resulting "transactions" may in their turn be whimsically categorized as: *Why Don't You* (covert command), *Yes But* (mutual frustration), *Uproar* (chaos), *Alcoholic* (I can't help my metabolic heredity), *Wooden Leg or Schlemiel* (I'm very sorry I'm so awkward), *Pirhana* (the group strips the cover-ups off one victim), PTA (parents against teachers against pupils and vice versa), and so on. Another frequent triangle with double arrows in all six directions is *Persecutor↔Rescuer↔Victim.* These games are segments of more complex and enduring patterns called *lifescripts,* which constitute each person's overall life plans and are used for the following purposes:

a.   *To reaffirm a position* (e.g., "All men are beasts").
b.   *To collect trading stamps* (e.g., *Brown*—"I am hurt and sulky;" *Blue*—"I have every right to be angry;" *Gray*—"you're driving me insane"). Accumulated "books of stamps" are traded in for presumed "Social Gains."
c.   To *get strokes*—i.e. handicap the opponents in the "game."
d.   To *stretch time* through various delays and rituals.
e.   And generally to *advance the script* by playing Cinderella, Ulysses, Oedipus, et al.

Such transactions may be exposed, interpreted, and counteracted in both dyadic or group sessions by the therapist or his surrogates. Groups are generally kept small (8–12) and may be entered only after each participant has clearly designated his therapeutic objectives and agreed to a formal *contract* (e.g., he must keep his job, control his drinking, adhere to the group mores, etc.) Meetings are held once or twice weekly and may be supplemented by individual interviews, designated readings, and ancillary assignments.

Berne and his trainees claim comparatively favorable and enduring results, and may well secure them in relatively intelligent, well integrated, and transactionally mobile patients whose prognosis had been rendered all the more favorable from the beginning by their possession of a sense of self-evaluative and transactional humor.

**Work Therapy,** properly prescribed and motivated, is widely utilized in socialist-oriented countries as a means of restoring physical well-being, self-respect, and social acceptance. However, psychiatrically indentured work may also be used to incarcerate and punish political dissidents (Z. Medvedev).

**Z-Therapy** (R. Zaslow) physically immobilizes a subject on the laps of eight "Z-assistants" with the subject's head near the therapist's abdomen. The subject is then plied with challenging questions such "Who's the boss?" "Why don't you respond?" to which appropriate answers must be given i.e., "You are!" "I love you!" literally on pain of having the subject's rib cage assaulted by a form of "tickling" which may become rough and traumatic. Predictable rage reactions ("A") reach peak ("B") experiences which purportedly "abolish negativism" and thereby "cure psychosomatic dysfunctions" ranging from childhood autism to adult schizophrenia.

### METAPSYCHOLOGIC AND RELIGIOUS MODALITIES

These offer an added parameter of reassuring faith in a superordinant system, (Ur III). The following are representative:

**Christian Science** (Mary Baker Eddy) asserts that Christian Science Truth can abolish diseases, all of which are conceived simply as "Mental Errors." Healing occurs through reading *Science and Health with Key to the Scriptures* with derived contemplation, or by personal or telepathic instruction. Church services include joint prayers and testimonials (Chapter 2).

**Faith Healings** have been practiced by *gurus, curanderos, shamans, hgangas* and other designated "medicine men" throughout history (Chapter 2). In indigenous cultural settings they have been demonstrably successful not only in relieving the psychic components of asthma, colitis, and similar somatic dysfunctions, but also in controlling highly disruptive behavior disorders such as *mal puesto* (a debilitating *hex*), *susto* (a severe stress reaction), and other aberrations ranging from paranoid panics to catatonic stupors. Western physicians had only their mystic reputations and placebos until quinine was shown to be the first effective drug, at about the middle of the last century, and all *medi*cations still *medi*ate the shared faiths of patient and prescriber (Chapter 12). With special ethnic groups, the physician may find it advantageous to collaborate with a folk healer to aid in therapy (P. Ruiz).

**Mystic Therapies.** Jan Ehrenwald, in his *Psychotherapy: Myth and Method*, records that Paracelsus extolled the healing power of religious beliefs; that Dr. Jenelm Digby's "powder of sympathy" was considered by kings and savants to be capable of healing battle wounds at a distance; that Ernst Cassirer held that "symbols, language, and myths are the only realities"; that Mesmer's doctrine of the therapeutic powers of animal magnetism was considered highly scientific by many authorities of his day; and that the eminent physicist Niels Bohr kept a horseshoe (vaginal symbol of Venus) nailed over his door "for good luck." Jan Ehrenwald cogently points out that all of us also live and benefit through "doctrinal compliance . . . with the myths" and accompanying customs of our culture, and that mental health is essentially (p. 156) "a syndrome of adaptation of a given individual in a given culture [i.e., mythology] at a given time."

**Religious Healings.** As associated with other Western faiths, these may range from local sacramental procedures for minor illness (e.g., clerical laying on of hands, sprinkling with holy water) to pilgrimages to holy shrines (Lourdes in France, Montserrat in Colombia)[3] where masses, prayers, priestly processions, and elaborate rituals hopefully invoke divine intervention for the correction of functional disabilities or the easing of terminal illnesses (Chapter 14).

As physical capacities fail and interpersonal alliances falter, faith in an omnipotently beneficent providence becomes increasingly necessary to existential serenity: ergo, physiology, psychiatry, and metapsychology can be effectively combined; indeed, in special instances, the author invites mutually respected priests, rabbis, or ministers to act as co-therapists (Ur III).

## Notes

1. Conceptually, dyadic therapies may also be considered as "group oriented," in that the patient brings into every session the surrogate influences of his family, friends, employers, and "significant others," whereas the therapist almost literally feels the presence of Freud, Adler, Glasser, Berne, or other chosen mentors.

2. S. Fenwick, J. Simon and L.L. Glass have published critiques of various idiosyncratic (Gk. *idios*-id-iotic) "Cults of the Self."

3. The author has witnessed self-styled "life-time cripples" abandon their crutches after a 3000 foot climb to this shrine.

*Chapter 12*

# PHARMACOLOGIC AND SOMATIC THERAPIES

These are frequently useful and at times essential in the management of extreme anxiety states, addictions, and psychotic disorders.

## ALCOHOLISM

The therapy of this clinically important syndrome comprises a transition from dyadic, behavioral and group to somatic modalities, and merits extended discussion.

**Experimental.** When administered to higher organisms, ethyl alcohol disorganizes complex behavior patterns, leaving simpler ones relatively intact. Correspondingly, when administered in moderate doses to animals rendered "experimentally neurotic" by being subjected to adaptational stresses (Chapter 5), alcohol literally dissolves inhibitions, phobias, compulsions, regressions and other complex "neurotic" reactions, permitting feeding, sex, and simpler manipulative behavior to reemerge. Many animals so relieved then prefer alcoholic to nonalcoholic drinks, thus developing an addiction that persists until their underlying neurosis is alleviated by individual retraining, group influences, or other procedures analogous to those employed in clinical therapies.[1]

Physiologic and psychologic studies in humans have similarly indicated that the ingestion of alcohol impairs adverse perceptions, clouds phobias, and dissolves inhibitions, and thereby permits previously repressed impulses to find release in action; ergo, patients who have found such surcease from interpersonal and social conficts—however illusory and evanescent—may continue to misuse alcohol to the point of addiction.

**Social Vectors.** Historically, men (and women) have nearly always and everywhere concocted and consumed various nepenthic substances such as mescal, psylocybin, aminata alkaloids, hashish, cocaine, and opiates as well as wines and liquors to attenuate inhibitions, relieve tensions, or release fantasies of mystic transcendence in religious rituals. Accordingly, in many cultures intoxication is accepted as mitigating censure for the expression of erotic (including homosexual) or aggressive conduct that would be condemned in a sober person. In our own society, an additional concept, although devoid of scientific validity,[2] has nevertheless found ready acceptance: namely, that alcoholism is always a metabolic "disease" for which the victim is not responsible—a rationalization that has seriously handicapped the thinking and therapy of 12 million alcoholic addicts, including 3 million teenagers, in this country alone.[3]

**Therapy of Alcoholism.** (a) *Acute.* Detoxification is best conducted in a setting where abstinence can be enforced, mild benzodiazepines administered for restlessness as necessary, and dietary and fluid balances restored. *Delerium tremens*, an agitated, hallucinatory furor that may follow the abrupt withdrawal of alcohol in severe intoxication is a relatively rare complication demanding parenteral sustenance, effective sedatives, and constant companionship to control delusional behavior. Alcoholic gastritis, neuritis, nephrosis, diabetes, and other systemic effects require appropriate medical care.

(b) *Comprehensive.* After 3 days of abstinence 0.5 g of Antabuse, or of the milder-acting deterrent Stopethyl, may be taken daily for several months, preferably in the presence of the spouse or other mentor, with the full understanding that even a single omission on any pretext undeniably signals an intent to resume drinking. However, as in all comprehensive therapy, such measures are merely the first stage of treatment. As soon as the patient's rapport has been secured and he has become more accessible and cooperative, every effort must be made to re-evoke his initiative, restore his strength, and renew his skills, (Ur I) and thus regain confidence and self-respect. The patient's sexual, marital, occupational, and other problems then require a tactful exploration of his personality development, his present goals and tribulations, his effective (normal), socially ineffective ("neurotic" or "sociopathic"), or bizarrely unrealistic (psychotic) conduct, the ways in which alcohol exacerbates his current diffi-culties, and how they might best be made amenable to various modalities of therapy. Retrospective reviews can be combined with gentle reasoning, personal guidance, and progressive social reorientations to alter childlike or escapist patterns of behavior that have long since lost their effectiveness, to revise goals and values, and adopt a more lastingly rewarding ("mature") style of life. The enlightened cooperation of family, friends, employer, organizations such as Alcoholics Anonymous, or other sources of effective support (v. self-help groups, Chapter 11) may, with the patient's assent, be secured and utilized to the fullest. By such means the patient's social needs will be strengthened by re-newed communal solidarity (Ur II) and cultural re-acceptance (Ur III)—a *sine qua non* of comprehensive treatment.

**Amytal Narcosis** (J. Masserman, 1955; L. Wolberg, 1978). The slow intravenous injection of from 0.1 gm. to 0.5 gm. of so-dium amytal in 10 percent solution to induce a state of semisom-nolence may calm excessive tensions and agitation, encourage communication, reveal repressed dependent, sexual, or aggres-sive conflicts for concurrent or later discussion, and enhance confidence in the therapist as a physician capable of utilizing medical measures when required. However, to avoid complica-tion, the possible side effects of intravenous barbiturates should be explained to the patient and his written permission for the interview obtained, including, whenever indicated, the presence of a witness.

**Antinarcotic Therapies** utilize various drugs: e.g., cyclazocine and naltrexone to counter opiate effects (Jaffe) or methadone (itself mildly addictive—Nyswander) to ease narcotic withdrawal. These procedures must always be supplemented by appropriate dyadic, group, or institutional therapies. The same is true of the spreading addiction to the smoking or parenteral abuse of cocaine, which now seriously affects over 8 million or more addicts in the U.S., with the added therapeutic difficulty that there are at present no effective substitute medications (R. Siegel).

**Biofeedback Techniques.** These employ electrocardiograms, sphygmomanometers, myograms, finger temperatures as skin resistance recorders (H.D. Kimmel), videotapes (I. Alger), and other devices by which subjects can be made technically aware of their somatic states at rest or under stress, and taught to control them through autosuggestion (T.X. Barber), relaxation (Jacobsen), meditation (B. Glueck), autohypnosis (H. Spiegel), or Yoga or Zen postures. Report on the successful alleviation of headaches (J.H. Budzynski), hypertension (A.K. Shapiro), hypotension (B.S. Brucher), wry neck (C. Cleeland), arthritic and back pains (R. Melzack, A.J. Nigel), Reynaud's disease (R.S. Surwit), spastic colitis (C.L. Birk) and epilepsy (M.D. Sterman) have lacked valid control studies (A.J. Yates). Other mechanical aides comprise devices such as wet-actuated electric stimulators to inhibit nocturnal enuresis, or a miniaturized metronome worn by a stutterer to help him synchronize his speech (C.L. Birk). More complicated devices can signal when patients smoke excessively (Azrin & Powell) or become too emotional in marital disputes (E.J. Thomas et al.).

**Dialysis** (H. Wagemaker). Sixteen weekly blood filtrations in a renal apparatus presumably remove circulating "schizophrenic toxins" such as, possibly, leu[5] or met[5] endorphines. As checked by the NIMH to control placebo and other effects (D. Leff), results are not encouraging.

**Electrocerebral Therapies.** These are employed in otherwise intractable psychotic states acutely dangerous to the patient or others. Their common feature is an intense physiochemical stimulation of the brain which causes muscular convulsions (reducible in intensity or eliminated by succinylcholine or other drugs) followed by a period of coma and progressive amnesia for preceding events. The biodynamic effects are highly complex mixtures of the following physical, psychologic, and social vectors.

*Physical.* The transcerebral currents stimulate the secretion of hypothalamic-pituitary and adrenal hormones, alter the balance of synaptic neuramines, create a period of unconsciousness, blunt memories of recent adversities, and presumably open neural circuits for reorganized learning.

*Psychologic.* Many patients, on later reflection, vividly recall feelings of terror preceding the onset of coma and/or during the postconvulsive state of confusion and bewilderment, and attribute an evoked "desire to get well" (i.e. to modify their psychotic behavior) to these highly aversive experiences. The induced forgetfulness of recent stresses and conflicts also helps clear the way for reconsideration, reorientation, readaptation, and rehabilitation under the therapist's guidance.

*Social.* More broadly, the reawakening after each treatment to a welcoming (and relieved) audience of physicians, nurses, and attendants has been described by some patients as a "symbolic rebirth" into a kindlier and more sympathetic world, to which the hospital furnishes a bridge of predominantly favorable influences.[4]

*Insulin Hypoglycemia; Indoklon Inhalations,* and other modalities of convulsive therapy must be modified for individual cases (i.e., brain damaged, aged), are subject to special complications, and are best employed in hospitals where medical and other emergency measures can be utilized.

In essence, shock therapies may be temporarily useful in relieving uncontrolled agitations or severe or suicidal depressions; however, they produce some loss of memory, effect no basic personality change unless supplemented by dynamically reorientative, reeducative, and rehabilitative therapies, and furnish no guarantee against the recurrence of acute or the persistence of chronic deviations of behavior (APA Task Force Report).

*Electrosleep* induced by a direct current of up to 20 volts from forehead to occiput, accompanied by an audio signal synchronized to the pulse, is a popular alternative to ECT in the USSR and India, but unsuccessful in controlled studies in the USA.

*Electrostimulation.* Direct pulses passed through electrodes implanted into the septum pellucidum, cerebellum, or elsewhere in the brain have been observed (R. Heath) to convert depressive affects into euphoric ones, inhibit epileptic discharges, and relieve neurotic and psychotic symptoms.

*Narcotherapy* utilizes the administration of various drugs (0.5-1.0 gm. in a 10% solution of amobarbital intravenously, supplemented orally by oxazepam, flurazepam, chloral hydrate, bromides or other sedatives) for protracted periods of sleep (H. Azima), occasionally lightened for food and hygiene by methylphenidate or other stimulants (L.A. Guill). The objectives are immediate relief from agitation, a prolonged regressive escape from external stresses, and receptivity to dependent guidance. Lesser intravenous doses and oral amobarbital, pentothal, or lysergic acid diethylamind (C. Dahlberg) disinhibit affective exploration and catharsis. See Amytal Narcosis, Sleep Therapy.

## PSYCHOPHARMACOLOGY[5]

Drugs useful to supplement more comprehensive programs of therapy are the following:

**Anxiolytic** (Table 12-1[6]) which help relieve trepidations, probably by attenuating bodily tensions. The principle short-

**TABLE 12-1**
**ANTIANXIETY AND HYPNOTIC DRUGS: PHARMACOKINETIC DATA**

| Drug | Absorption: t max hours (Relative Rate) | Most Significant Biologically Active Compounds in Blood | Mean (Range) Half-life hours | Volume of Distribution L/kg | Clearance ml/min/kg |
|---|---|---|---|---|---|
| BENZODIAZEPINES | | | | | |
| *Compounds With Active Metabolites* | | | | | |
| Chlordiazepoxide [Libritabs, Librium] | 0.5-4 (Intermediate) | Chlordiazepoxide Desmethylchlor- diazepoxide | 9.9 (8-24) (24-96) | 0.3 ± 0.03 | 0.37 ± 0.06 |
| Clorazepate [Tranxene] | 1-2 (Fast) | Desmethyldiazepam | (50-100) | 0.93-1.27 | |
| Diazepam [Valcaps, Valium, Valrelease] | 1.5-2 (Fast) | Diazepam Desmethyldiazepam | (27-37) (50-100) | 0.95-2 0.93-1.27 | 0.38 ± 0.06 |
| Flurazepam [Dalmane] | 0 5-2 (Intermediate) | Desalkylflurazepam | (74-160)* | 3.4 | |
| Halazepam [Paxipam] | 1-3 (Intermediate) | Halazepam Desmethyldiazepam | 14 (50-100) | 0.93-1.27 | |
| Prazepam [Centrax] | 6 (Slow) | Desmethyldiazepam | (50-100) | 0.93-1.27 | |
| *Compounds With Weakly Active or Inactive Metabolites* | | | | | |
| Alprazolam [Xanax] | 1-2 (Fast) | Alprazolam | 12.1 (11.1-19) | | |
| Clonazepam [Clonopin] | 1-2 (Intermediate) | Clonazepam | (18-50) | | |
| Lorazepam [Ativan] | 2 (Intermediate) | Lorazepam | 15 (8-25) | 1.0-1.3 | 0.7-1.2 |
| Oxazepam [Serax] | 1-4 (Slow) | Oxazepam | (5-15) | 0.6-2 | 0.9-2 |
| Temazepam [Restoril] | 2-3 (Slow) | Temazepam | 14.7 (8-38) | 1.4-1.5 | 1.1-1.4 |
| Triazolam [Halcion] | 1.3 (Fast) | Triazolam | 2.6 (1.7-5.2) | 0.8-1.3 | 3.7-10.6 |
| *Investigational Agents* | | | | | |
| Flunitrazepam [Rohypnol] | IV USE | Flunitrazepam | 20 | | |
| Midazolam | IV USE | Midazolam | 2.5 ± 2.17 | 1.72 ± 0.05 | 8.1 |
| BARBITURATES | | | | | |
| Butabarbital [Butisol] | | Butabarbital | 100 (66-140) | | |
| Phenobarbital | 6-18 | Phenobarbital | 79 (53-118) | | |
| Mephobarbital [Mebaral] | 6-18 | Mephobarbital Phenobarbital | 79 (53-118) | | |
| Amobarbital [Amytal] | 2 | Amobarbital | 25 (16-40) | | |

**TABLE 12-1 (continued)**
**ANTIANXIETY AND HYPNOTIC DRUGS: PHARMACOKINETIC DATA**

| Drug | Absorption: t max hours (Relative Rate) | Most Significant Biologically Active Compounds in Blood | Mean (Range) Half-life hours | Volume of Distribution L/kg | Clearance ml/min/kg |
|---|---|---|---|---|---|
| **BARBITURATES** | | | | | |
| Pentobarbital [Nembutal] | 2 | Pentobarbital | (15-50) | | |
| Secobarbital [Seconal] | 2 | Secobarbital | 28 (15-40) | | |
| **NONBENZODIAZEPINE-NONBARBITURATES** | | | | | |
| *Antianxiety Agents* | | | | | |
| Hydroxyzine [Atarax, Orgatrax, Vistaril] | | Hydroxyzine | (2.5-3.4) | | |
| Meprobamate [Equanil, Mepro-span, Miltown] | 2-3 | Meprobamate | (10-24) | | |
| Propranolol [Inderal] (Investigational use) | 1-3 | Propranolol Hydroxypropranolol | 3.9 ± 0.4 | 3.9 ± 0.6 | 12 ± 3 |
| *Hypnotic Agents (prescription)* | | | | | |
| Chloral Hydrate | | Trichloroethanol | (4-9.5) | | |
| Ethchlorvynol [Placidyl] | | Ethchlorvynol | (10-25) | | |
| Ethinamate [Valmid] | | Ethinamate | 2.5 | | |
| Glutethimide [Doriden] | | Glutethimide | (5-22) | | |
| Methaqualone [Mequin, Parest, Quaalude] | | Methaqualone | (19-41) | | |
| Methyprylon [Noludar] | | Methyprylon | 4 | | |
| Paraldehyde [Paral] | 0.5-1 | Paraldehyde | 7.4 (3.4-9.8) | 0.8-1.2 | |
| *Hypnotic Agents (anti-histamines [nonprescription])* | | | | | |
| Diphenhydramine [Sominex Formula 2] | | Diphenhydramine | | | |
| Doxylamine [Unisom] | | Doxylamine | 9.3 (4-12) | | |
| Pyrilamine [Nervine, Nytol, Sleep-Eze, Sominex] | | Pyrilamine | | | |

*Mean half-life (hours): young males, 74; elderly males, 160; young females, 90; elderly females, 120 acting drugs and their standard doses are triazolam (Halcion, 0.25-0.50 mgm.) and oxazepam (Serax, 15-30 mgm). Flurazepam (Dalmane, 15-30 mgm.) induces sleep, but often with diurnal drowsiness. Alprazolam (Xanax), chlorazepate (Tranxene) and other "tranquilizers" are not demonstrably more effective; however, Buspirone at 15 to 20 mgm/d may have fewer interdrug, addictive and withdrawal effects as compared with the benzodiazepenes.

**Drugs for Affective Disorders (Table 12-2).** These are of questionable utility for the frustrations, disappointments, and reactive hypothymias of life; however, in the severe melancholias or manic-depressive cycles of possible genetic-neurochemical origin, their administration, after a cumulative period of 10–21 days, may help improve appetite and sleep, restore energy, favor rapport, and modify morbid or suicidal preoccupations—although with variable gastrointestinal, genitourinary, visual, or other side effects. The drugs in common use, with few demonstrable differences in action, are imimpramine (Tofranil), desipramine (Norpramin), doxapine (Sinequan), amitryptoline (Elavil), and protryptaline (Vivactil), prescribed in lesser doses to the elderly. If these are found ineffective, monoamino oxidase (MAO) inhibitors i.e.: phenelzine (Nardil), tranylcypromine (Parnate), or similar drugs that prevent the oxidation of stimulating (*energic*) catechol or indol cerebral amines, may be utilized, but only if tyramine or other amine-containing foods (cheeses, liver, herring, etc.) and beers and wines are eliminated from the diet. Recently introduced antidepressants (Maprotyline, Trazodone, Buproprione, Nomaphesin) with differing chemical structures and central effects are claimed to act more rapidly and with fewer disadvantages, but reports as to their comparative usefulness vary.

*Lithium Carbonate* is currently favored to prevent or control recurrent paranoid or manic episodes, but because of its potential cardiac, hepatic, and renal toxicity the dosage must be carefully monitored as to salt intake and by biweekly and later monthly laboratory assays to keep the blood content between 0.7

## TABLE 12-2
## DRUGS USED IN AFFECTIVE DISORDERS

| Classification | Drug | Aliphatic Amine Type | Sedative Activity | Anti-cholinergic Activity | Adult (Outpatient) Daily Dose Range During Initial Treatment* (mg) |
|---|---|---|---|---|---|
| **ANTIDEPRESSANTS** | | | | | |
| TRICYCLIC COMPOUNDS | | | | | |
| Dibenzazepines | Desipramine Norpramin (Merrell Dow) Pertofrane (USV) | Secondary | Minimal | Minimal | 75**-150 |
| | Imipramine Imavate (Robins) SK-Pramine (Smith Kline & French) Tofranil (Geigy) | Tertiary | Intermediate | Intermediate | 75**-150 |
| | Trimipramine Surmontil (Ives) | Tertiary | Maximal | Intermediate | 75**-150 |
| Dibenzocyclo-heptadienes | Protriptyline Vivactil (Merck Sharp & Dohme) | Secondary | Minimal | Intermediate | 15**-40 |
| | Nortriptyline Aventyl (Lilly) Pamelor (Sandoz) | Secondary | Intermediate | Minimal | 20**-100 |
| | Amitriptyline Elavil (Merck Sharp & Dohme) Endep (Roche) Enovil (Hauck) SK-Amitriptyline (Smith Kline & French) | Tertiary | Maximal | Maximal | 75**-150 |
| Dibenzoxepin | Doxepin Adapin (Pennwalt) Sinequan (Roerig) | Tertiary | Maximal | Maximal | 75**-150 |
| Dibenzoxazepine | Amoxapine Asendin (Lederle) | Not Applicable | Minimal | Minimal | 75**-400 |
| TETRACYCLIC COMPOUND | | | | | |
| | Maprotiline Ludiomil (Ciba) | Secondary | Intermediate | Intermediate | 75**-150 |
| TRIAZOLOPYRIDINE COMPOUND | | | | | |
| | Trazodone Desyrel (Mead Johnson) | Not Applicable | Intermediate | Minimal | 75**-300 |
| MONOAMINE OXIDASE INHIBITORS | | | | | |
| Hydrazines | Isocarboxazid Marplan (Roche) | | | | 20-40 |
| | Phenelzine Nardil (Parke, Davis) | | | | 45-120 |
| Nonhydrazine | Tranylcypromine Parnate (Smith Kline & French) | | | | 20-50 |

| Classification | Drug | Aliphatic Amine Type | Sedative Activity | cholinergic Activity | Adult (Outpatient) Daily Dose Range During Initial Treatment* (mg) |
|---|---|---|---|---|---|
| **ANTIMANIC** | Lithium | | | | 600-2100 (Initial) |
| | Cibalith-S (Ciba) | | | | 900-1200 (Maintenance) |
| | Eskalith (Smith Kline & French) | | | | |
| | Lithane (Miles) | | | | |
| | Lithobid (Ciba) | | | | |
| | Lithonate (Rowell) | | | | |
| | Lithotabs (Rowell) | | | | |

*Initial treatment (treatment of the initial phase) is regarded as the 4- to 8-week period until the patient becomes nearly symptom-free; treatment usually is instituted with the smaller dose of the range listed and gradually increased to the larger dose, if required (see the following footnote). Doses larger than those listed often are required in severely depressed inpatients or in drug-resistant patients (see the evaluations). Continuation treatment at the optimal daily dose (or somewhat less) determined during initial treatment usually is then instituted for a period of approximately 20 consecutive weeks. Controlled studies are in progress to determine if maintenance treatment is indicated beyond continuation treatment, usually at a lower daily dose than that utilized during continuation treatment.

**One useful schedule that lessens the intensity of undesirable sedative, hypotensive, and anticholinergic effects initially in outpatients and makes dosage adjustment easier follows: Imipramine (or an equivalent dose of the antidepressants other than the monoamine oxidase inhibitors and lithium) 25 mg twice daily for three days, 50 mg twice daily for three days, and 75 mg twice daily for the next ten days. A minimum of five days between dosage adjustments may be more appropriate in the elderly, the debilitated, or patients with cardiac disease and may be particularly desirable to avoid undue sedation and hypotension that may result in injury. (If insomnia is prominent, it may be preferable to give the initial daily amount as a single dose at bedtime to obtain the full benefit of sedation and minimize functional impairment and drowsiness during the day.) After two to three weeks of therapy, a single daily dose is commonly given at bedtime. If limited benefit is observed by the third week, the daily dose is increased, usually weekly, until satisfactory improvement, intolerable adverse reactions, or the recommended maximum dose is reached (see the evaluations).

to 1.2mEq/liter, since levels above 1.75mEq may cause serious organic dysfunctions, delirium, and death.

**Antipsychotic Drugs** (Table 12-3) are utilized to diminish delusional or destructive behavior, improve personal hygiene, and render the patient more amenable to dyadic and group therapies. Standard are chlorpromazine (Thorazine), and thioridazine (Mellaril). For more rapid action, haloperidol (Haldol) or thifluperazine (Stelazine) may be injected intramuscularly; fluphenazine decanoate (Prolixin) may be similarly administered for prolonged absorption in uncooperative patients. Unfortunately the neurochemical action of the phenothiazines and butyrophenones in blocking dopamine and other cerebral receptors may also cause hypotension, gastrointestinal, and

**TABLE 12-3**
**ANTIPSYCHOTIC DRUGS**

| Drug | Chemical Classification | Therapeutically Equivalent Oral Dose (mg) | Effects | | |
|---|---|---|---|---|---|
| | | | Sedation | Autonomic[1] | Extrapyramidal Reactions[2] |
| Fluphenazine Permitil (Schering) Prolixin (Squibb) | Phenothiazine: Piperazine Compound | 2 | +/++ | + | +++ |
| Haloperidol Haldol (McNeil) | Butyrophenone | 2 | + | + | +++ |
| Thiothixene Navane (Roerig) | Thioxanthene | 4 | + | + | +++ |
| Trifluoperazine Stelazine (Smith Kline & French) | Phenothiazine: Piperazine Compound | 5 | ++ | + | +++ |
| Perphenazine Trilafon (Schering) | Phenothiazine: Piperazine Compound | 8 | +/++ | + | +++ |
| Loxapine Loxitane (Lederle) | Dibenzoxazepine | 10 | ++ | +/++ | ++/+++ |
| Molindone Moban (Endo) | Dihydroindolone | 10 | ++ | ++ | ++/+++ |
| Piperacetazine Quide (Merrell Dow) | Phenothiazine: Piperidine Compound | 10 | ++ | + | ++ |
| Prochlorperazine Compazine (Smith Kline & French) | Phenothiazine: Piperazine Compound | 15 | ++ | + | +++ |
| Acetophenazine Tindal (Schering) | Phenothiazine: Piperazine Compound | 20 | ++ | + | +++ |
| Carphenazine Proketazine (Wyeth) | Phenothiazine: Piperazine Compound | 25 | ++ | + | +++ |
| Triflupromazine Vesprin (Squibb) | Phenothiazine: Aliphatic Compound | 25 | +++ | ++/+++ | ++ |
| Mesoridazine Serentil (Boehringer Ingelheim) | Phenothiazine: Piperidine Compound | 50 | +++ | ++ | + |
| Chlorpromazine Thorazine (Smith Kline & French) | Phenothiazine: Aliphatic Compound | 100 | +++ | ++/+++ | ++ |
| Chlorprothixene Taractan (Roche) | Thioxanthene | 100 | +++ | +++ | +/++ |
| Thioridazine Mellaril (Sandoz) | Phenothiazine: Piperidine Compound | 100 | +++ | ++/+++ | + |
| INVESTIGATIONAL Pimozide Orap (McNeil) | Diphenylbutylpiperidine | | + | + | ++ |
| Clozapine Leponex | Dibenzodiazepine | | +++ | +++ | +/- |

[1]Alpha antiadrenergic and anticholinergic effects
[2]Excluding tardive dyskinesia which appears to be produced to the same degree and frequency by all agents with equieffective antipsychotic doses

urinary dysfunctions, impotence, and disorders of muscular control such as diplopia, restless movements (akathisia), muscular tremors and rigidities (Parkinsonism), oral, lingual and facial grimacing (tardive dyskinesia) and other variably serious effects not always reversible by reduced dosage, or by medicaments such as Cogentin and Artane (*vi*).

*Sleep Therapy* (J. Klaesi), popular in the Soviet Union, employs 3–7 days of narcosis induced by combinations of phenothiazines, barbiturates, scopalamine, and other hypnotics for both neurotic and psychotic disorders, with partial waking for feeding and elimination, and precautions against aspiration and drug reactions. Paradoxically, Einar Kringlen of Oslo recommends several days and nights of sleep deprivation as an effective therapy for depressions.

### Miscellaneous

*Methylphenidate* (Ritalin) which usually acts as a stimulant has nevertheless been found useful in controlling the behavior of constitutionally overactive children.

*Opiade peptides and enkaphalins,* naturally occurring neurotransmitters which act like opiates, have been tried in alleviating the "cerebral pain" in depressive or catatonic states, but with dubious results.

*Lysergic acid diethylamide (LSD)* has been reported to expedite imagery and communication in withdrawn patients, but with the recurrence of hallucinatory experiences and other clinical risks.

*Artane* 4–12 mg daily or Cogentin 1–4 mg/d may counter the muscular rigidities of Parkinsonism, and propanolol or Nadolol 30–80 mg/d may be helpful in the restlessness of akathisia.

In essence, the use of drugs in psychiatry requires as thorough a knowledge of chemistry, neurophysiology, and pharmacology and as much care in clinical observation, dosage, coordination with other therapies and follow-up as in any other branch of medicine, as further illustrated in the following chapter.

## NOTES

1. Demonstated by the author (1946) and confirmed by Jacobsen in Copenhagen, Shankar in Vienna, and others. Dr. Shankar repeated my experiments and recorded them in a color and sound film available from Pfizer Laboratories (Masserman, 1955).

2. Masserman, *Alcohol, Diseases or Dis-ease?* 1961. Peele, S, *Addiction: a Comprehensive Theory*, 1985.

3. At additional costs of 43 billion dollars and 20,000 deaths annually (U.S. Dept. of Alcohol Studies). For more salutary effects, physicians may prescribe sedative ("sitting") or hypnotic (sleeping) drugs to patients to blunt disturbing perceptions, diminish unnecessary fears, and furnish temporary but welcome relief—always with proper precautions against inducing addictions and withdrawal syndromes.

4. J. Lanbaurn and D. Gill reported that in 16 patients "simulated ECT" (preliminary relaxing and anesthetic procedures without shock currents, followed by the routine aftercare) produced favorable results equal to those in 16 patients given electroshocks.

5. For a more detailed discussion of the special indications, actions, and clinical precautions in the use of psychoactive drugs, see Masserman, 1980.

6. Tables 12-1, 12-2 and 12-3 are reproduced from the Fifth Edition of *AMA Drug Evaluations* by permission of the American Medical Association.

*Chapter 13*

# PSYCHIATRIC DISORDERS IN PHYSICALLY ILL PATIENTS[1]

Psychiatric symptomatology may complicate the diagnosis and treatment of a patient's serious physical illness; conversely, and more frequently, physical symptoms may obscure a concurrent mental disorder.

Although many psychiatric symptoms and syndromes are produced directly by physical illness [e.g. the anxiety of hyperthyroidism, the protean effects of the misuse of cocaine (Gold & Verebey), delirium with infections, high fever, or the complications of surgery], emotional reactions to physical illness (e.g., depressions, panic states) are frequently either overlooked or too readily dismissed. Their clinically important interrelationships are discussed below.

## PSYCHIATRIC MANIFESTATIONS OF PHYSICAL ILLNESS

The great physicians of the past were aware of the psychiatric accompaniments of physical illness. In the description of the disease that bears his name, R. Graves wrote about the psychoneurotic symptomatology of thyrotoxicosis. In the first account of neurodermatitis in 1891, L. Brocque and L. Jacquet stated that anxiety was a prominent feature. W. Osler emphasized the psychiatric symptomatology produced by many diseases and insisted on care for their attendant psychic distress. However, in some quarters there are still inadequate provisions for the psychiatric therapy of physically ill patients, attributable in part to the reductionism of specialization, the apparent decline in humanism, and to persistent concepts of psycho-somatic dualism.

## THE BRAIN

The psychiatric symptomatology produced by disease of the brain may be the patient's presenting syndrome. Such personality changes as brooding, irritability, or suspiciousness may herald the onset of a brain tumor. When these signs are hidden by the mask of depression, the underlying malignant process may not be apparent until moderately late in the course of the illness. Except for metastatic disease, the development of psychiatric symptoms produced by brain tumors is seldom abrupt and generally appears as an exaggeration of premorbid personality traits. The fairly sudden development of a hypomanic or manic condition in a middle-aged patient with no previous history of such behavior should alert the clinician to the possibility of an organic condition. Depressive symptomatology is seen frequently in patients with brain tumors; generally, the most prominent feature is retardation rather than marked lowering of mood or somatic symptomatology, except for headache. Localization of the tumor influences symptomatology (Table 13-1.).

With epileptic patients, diagnostic and treatment errors are made in two totally different directions. So much emphasis may be placed on a slight abnormality in the EEG that the patient's emotional illness is falsely attributed to an epileptic disturbance and he receives epileptic medications rather than needed psychotherapy. Conversely, because epilepsy usually makes its appearance in adolescence or young adulthood when the person is undergoing rapid physical and psychological changes, the symptomatology may be attributed to the stresses of that time of life and the diagnosis and treatment of epilepsy overlooked. The possibility of drug abuse further complicates diagnosis (Table 13-2).

## TABLE 13-1
## SYMPTOMS OF BRAIN TUMORS

| Site | Symptoms |
|------|----------|
| Frontal lobes | Personality change |
| | Frontal lobe syndrome—childishness, inattention, loss of judgment |
| Temporal lobe | Insidious personality change |
| | Anxiety, irritability |
| | Visual or auditory hallucinations |
| Parietal lobe | Disturbances of sensation |
| | Focal seizures |
| | Anxiety, low tolerance to frustration |
| Occipital lobe | Headaches |
| | Visual disturbances |
| Pituary | Decreased (occasionally increased) libido |
| | Disturbances of body image |
| Floor of III Ventricle | Disturbed hypothalamic-pituitary function and manifest anxiety |

## TABLE 13-2
## PSYCHIATRIC SYMPTOMS ASSOCIATED
## WITH SOME EPILEPTIC DISORDERS

| Disorder | Symptoms |
|----------|----------|
| Temporal lobe epilepsy | Confusion, negativism, automatisms |
| | Hallucinations (visual, auditory, haptic) |
| | Poor impulse control |
| Atonic seizure | Disturbance of consciousness |
| | Fainting, aberrant behavior |
| Episodic dyscontrol | Assaultiveness |
| Syndrome | Pathological intoxication |
| | History of automobile accidents |

## ENDOCRINE DISORDERS

Because hormones exert their effects on many organs and systems, the manifestations of endocrine disease can be numerous, vague, and often bizarre. Endocrine dysfunctions usually appear gradually; consequently, they are difficult to diagnose in their early stages, and the patient with ill-defined symptomatology may easily be labeled "neurotic." Thus, many patients may be perceived as being only psychiatrically ill and their endocrine diseases not fully evaluated. The appearance of depression is particularly confusing; more than any other psychiatric diagnosis it is applied to patients with endocine disorders. Even more commonly, however, the endocrine patient's emotional distress is not regarded as significant and he or she does not receive needed psychiatric treatment (Table 13-3).

### TABLE 13-3
### SYMPTOMS OF ENDOCRINE DISORDERS

| Disorders | Symptoms |
|-----------|----------|
| Hyperthyroidism | Manifest anxiety with many physical symptoms |
| | Palpitations, restlessness, sweating |
| | Depression in later stages |
| | Psychosis |
| Hypothyroidism | Generalized discomfort |
| | Apathy, difficulty concentrating |
| | Depression |
| | "Myxedema madness" with psychotic symptoms |
| Hypercortisolism (pituitary or adrenal disease or induced) | Early onset of psychiatric symptoms |
| | Irritability and lability of mood |
| | Occasionally euphoria but depression is common |
| | Body image disturbances |
| | Steroid psychosis |
| Hypocortisolism (pituitary or adrenal) | Weakness, fatigue, lack of initiative, negativism, depression |
| | Organic brain syndromes late |

| | |
|---|---|
| Hyperparathyroidism | Weakness, lassitude, dysphoria |
| | Depression |
| | Organic mental disorders especially delirium |
| Hypoparathyroidism | Weakness, fatigue, irritability |
| | Tetany may be mistaken for conversion |
| Hyperinsulinism | Weakness, anxiety, confusion |
| | Fainting |
| | Appears to be "neurotic" |
| Hyperestrogenemia | Depression |
| Hypoestrogenemia | Vasomotor distress |
| | Affective lability with tearfulness |
| | Depression |
| | Passivity, low sex drive |
| | Turner's Syndrome (retarded deveopment) |
| Hyperandrogenemia | In males, irritability and insomnia |
| | In females, increased sex drive |
| Hypoandrogenemia | Kleinfelter's Syndrome (feminization) |
| | Decreased sex drive in males and females |
| | Irritability, episodic depression |

## REACTIONS TO PHYSICAL ILLNESS

Physical as well as mental illnesses occur in a setting which includes the environment, acculturation, learning, the family, and available social and economic resources, along with the significance of the sick role and attitudes toward medical care. Since physical illness is the most common threat to well-being in our modern world, it evokes basic emotional responses. Anxiety, regression, depression, grief, and denial are the fundamental reactions, often combined, as outlined below.

**Anxiety.** Anxiety springs from concerns about diagnosis and prognosis, problems associated with obtaining medical care and the rigors of treatment, and the effects of illness on functioning. Displacement of anxiety occurs with medical illness and hospitalization. A typical example is the cardiac patient who expresses concern about the accuracy of diagnosis and the expense of hospitalization rather than about stressful situations at home and at work which preceded the onset of the illness and threaten to complicate convalescence. Displacement of anxiety to specific bodily functions can also intensify symptoms.

**Regression.** Since anxiety has a signal function indicating that well-being is threatened, it leads to preoccupation with the self. The regression usually includes some limitation of physical activity, behavioral changes, and increased dependency with its implicit and explicit demands on others. Complaining, self-centered attitudes evoke responses which may be either overtly or covertly hostile. Physicians, nurses, and the family become concerned because they fear that the patient will persist in a stage of helpless dependency and not cooperate with therapy —all of which can retard convalescence and exacerbate interpersonal difficulties. In most cases the regression is transient; however, the resulting interpersonal tensions between the patient, family, and the health care team may persist as distrust and resentment.

**Grief.** As described by J. Bowlby, the grief reaction moves through three major phases—protest, despair, and detachment. Patients may respond initially to loss of comfort, function, and freedom by resistance to diagnostic procedures or treatment initiatives. In the protest phase of a grief reaction, patients may be hypercritical of physicians, other members of the health care team, and of their families. As this gives ground to pessimism or despair, disturbed sleep and appetite, an impaired self-image, and social withdrawal become evident, although some patients eventually accept the illness and determine to resolve attendant problems more realistically.

**Denial.** In its severe forms, denial is probably the most pathological reaction to illness. Excessive denial is indicative of a diminished ego strength which requires negation of the threat to the integrity of the organism. Excessive denial precludes agreement between the patient and the physician about the severity of the illness so that cooperation is replaced by dissension. J. L. Titchner and M. Levine found that such reactions were often responsible for delaying surgery until cure was no longer possible.

**Depression.** Diagnosing depression in physically ill patients can be difficult, because such somatic symptoms as loss of appetite or insomia may be caused by the illness or masked by it. Patients who have a family history of affective disorder are at higher risk than others, but virtually anyone who endures a major illness for an extended period of time is likely to become depressed and to need treatment. The distinction between depression and a normal grief reaction can be difficult. Self-recrimination, self-destructive thoughts, and suicidal ideation are not typical symptoms of a grief reaction but are reasonalby reliable indicators of depression. Depression also decreases tolerance for pain and other symptoms, thus complicating therapy and inhibiting recovery.

### TREATMENT

Three general principles apply to the treatment of psychiatric disorders in physically ill patients.

First, diagnostic efforts should include attempts to understand the patient as a person, to assess risk and vulnerability, and to identify psychiatric symptoms and syndromes (Chapters 3, 4).

Second, the presence of physical illness does not preclude psychiatric treatment for the patient's emotional distress or mental disorder. Too frequently, psychiatric treatment is relegated to a secondary position and sometimes either stopped or postponed until the patient recovers from the physical illness. True, diagnostic differentiation of the role of the physical illness, and its treatments may pose some difficulties for the psychiatrist working with the physically ill patient, but this does not necessarily bar psychotherapy, which can reduce the length of hospitalization, morbidity and mortality (Chapters 5, 6).

Third, the psychiatrist should not overlook the need for rehabilitation and resocialization programs for physically ill patients with psychiatric symptomatology (Chapters 8–12).

The major psychotherapeutic objectives are: 1) to provide encouragement; 2) to deal with the effects on the patient and the family; 3) to focus on both the direct and indirect effects of the illness, its prognosis, and possible long-term changes in life style and functioning; and 4) to obtain compliance with medical and surgical treatments and rehabilitation.

Special techniques for the seriously ill are: 1) to employ a warmer, more empathetic attitude than one does customarily; 2) to employ active psychotherapy; 3) to deal directly with fears and adverse fantasies; 4) to clarify misunderstandings about the bodily functions affected; and 5) to recognize that some degree of denial may be a necessary defense against hopelessness, but that excessive lack of realism is usually counterproductive.

For patients with chronic or recurring illnesses, psychotherapy should also be directed toward accepting the necessary restrictions of activity and the rigors of treatment in a lifelong perspective, with reassurances that their doctors will not abandon them.

The treatment of grief requires a display of patience, a tolerant attitude, and a willingness to listen to the patient during the protest phase. During despair, the psychiatrist has to probe for and to urge the patient to discuss feelings, and fears with all their ambivalence and uncertainty. In the detachment phase, offering support and reassurance is all that is necessary. As a general rule, the more serious the loss, the longer will it take for the patient to move through the phases of a grief reaction. It is helpful to assure the patient's family and one's colleagues that protest and despair are normal phases of a response to illness. But when the grief reaction is severe and prolonged, the physically ill patient usually needs intensive psychotherapy focused on deprivation hostility, ambivalence, and grief.

**Medications.** When the physically ill patient's condition permits, the judicious use of medications for creating emotional distress and mental symptomatology may be necessary components of the total program. For example, propanalol substantially reduces the anxiety associated with thyrotoxicosis or pheochromocytoma, haloperidol controls the manic behavior of a patient with a metastatic brain tumor, and chlorpromazine quiets the delirious patient. Such short acting benzodiazepine anxiolytics as oxazepam or lorazepam are usually the agents of choice for the physically ill patient, since their metabolism does not involve demethylation by the cytochrome P-450 system in the liver. Also, there is little danger of a drug withdrawal reaction when they are used for only a short period of time.

For the treatment of depression, the psychiatrist can recommend such tricyclic medications as imipramine, doxepin, or trazodone provided that the anticholinergic and cardiovascular side effects, will not be detrimental (Chapter 12). Because it has a rapid onset of action and few adverse effects other than sedation and ataxia, alprazolam may be the antidepressant of choice for physically ill patients. Generally, the monoamine oxidase inhibitors are to be avoided. For psychotic or delirious patients, antipsychotic medications such as chlorpromazine and haloperidol are necessary; in extreme depressions, electroconvulsive treatment can be life saving. Prompt treatment is imperative because the psychotic state usually interferes with needed medical or surgical treatments.

In all cases, when working with physically ill patients, the psychiatrist should discuss the use of medications with the presiding physician or surgeon and be alert to the possibility of drug interactions.

**Rehabilitation and Resocialization.** These programs should be aimed toward increasing activity mentally, physically and socially, particularly during convalescence. Assistance from the clergy, physical and recreational therapists, and from specialists in rehabilitation medicine can be directly helpful to the patient and reassuring to the family.

**The Patient's Family.** Family members often fear that the mental symptoms in the physically ill signify increased severity, long-term impairment, or a poor prognosis, and begin to feel helpless, guilty, and/or hostile to the patient or the medical team. The psychiatrist can allay fears, supply information about the illness, clarify distortions, and provide support for all concerned.

Finally, not only do patients and their families benefit, but the psychiatrist increases his colleagues' respect for him as a member of the medical team.

## NOTE

1.  The author is deeply indebted to John J. Schwab, M.D. and Clifford C. Kuhn, M.D., respectively Chairman and Vice Chairman of the Department of Behavioral Sciences at the University of Louisville for furnishing the medical data for this chapter.

# Chapter 14

# THERAPY AT VARIOUS AGES

## REVIEW OF PRINCIPLES

Most human beings serve others "in-tuitively" (inwardly taught) well, since children in a civilized society must learn to do so, else suffer early penalties. To implement this latent empathy, the psychotherapist's professional education (L., *e-duce*, to lead out) should develop his special capacities to help those who appeal to him for solace and comfort by alleviating their physical, social, or philosophic Ur tribulations as follows (Chapters 1, 2, 5, 6):

**Ur I: First, by Improving Function and Allaying Pain and Fear.** Anxiolytic and antidepressive medications (Chapter 12) are useful while underlying organic illnesses are also treated. As examples, gastric or duodenal ulcers require antacids, antispasmodics, and proper diets; the lassitude and fatigue of the anemic will respond to supplemental vitamin $B_{12}$ and other hematopoetic measures, the sword-of-Damocles apprehensive restlessness of the latent epileptic will diminish under anti-ictal medication sufficient to control his seizures, and so on for other somatic illnesses as described in Chapter 13.

**Ur II: Next, the Therapist must Help Rebuild the Patient's Interpersonal Securities.** Whatever his complaints, consciously or not, the patient comes to the therapist much as a hurt and frightened child appeals to his parents for individual, devoted, and seemingly unselfish care, or as an ally against a disappointing or hostile world. It is therefore essential to learn what familial, economic, occupational, or other life stresses may have occasioned his somatic and social difficulties, as outlined in chapter 3 and 4. This preliminary survey will often reveal direct relationships between intercurrent life events and easily recognizable psychiatric syndromes. Therapy can then be more effectively directed toward familial, social, occupational, esthetic, and creative readaptations (Chapters 5 through 14).

**Ur III: Third, the Therapist can Help Restore the Patient's Necessary Faiths in a Mundane or Cosmic Order.** If indicated, this can be done by collaborating with a minister, rabbi, or priest incidentally earning reciprocal respect and cooperation from men of the cloth.

Effective implementation of these Ur objectives in therapy has sometimes been compared to a game of chess: the principles governing the opening and closing moves can be fairly clearly stated, but the maneuvers in between must ever be determined by the talent, insight, and forethought of each player in dealing with the other's moves. Accordingly, there are few rules that will guarantee success in every or even any instance, but these generalizations may be helpful:

Therapy cannot be determined by a one- or two-word DSM III or DRG[1] label. Instead, the therapist must understand the nature of the patient's motives, tribulations, the effective ("normal"), socially deviant ("neurotic"), or culturally dereistic ("psychotic") ways he tries to deal with them, and the relative accessibility of these patterns of behavior to the therapeutic influences outlined in Chapters 5–13.

It is true that the patient's conduct has evolved from his previous life experiences, but those cannot be relived and changed; instead, the patient's *reactions* to his past should be explored and evaluated primarily to clarify their currently adverse but alterable residues. In general, brief, direct, and effective therapy concentrates on the patient's *real* and *present* problems and their practical solutions. *Progress consists of abandoning patterns that are no longer adequate and exploring and adopting new ones that are more personally and socially profitable.*

Rarely, however, should the therapist furnish arbitrary directions as to the selection of a career, conception or adoption of a child, initiating or stopping of a divorce action, or other major changes. If the patient is helped to see clearly the alternatives and consequences of his behavior, he will not need such advice; if he follows it blindly, dubiously, or resentfully, his actions are quite likely to circumvent or vitiate its intent—and the therapist will, quite justifiably, be blamed for the results. The patient's confidences, of course, are never violated, but this does not exclude conferences with—or concurrent psychotherapy of—his friends, family, employer, or other persons who may be contributing to or sharing his difficulties.

The principles reviewed above outline the rationale and goals of therapy, but their application must take account of multiple clinical contingencies: the patient's constitutional predispositions, age and sex, the type, intensity, and duration of the maladaptations, the economic, social, and cultural milieu, and many other factors. This complexity has led some practitioners to declare that "psychotherapy is an *art* rather than a science" —an aphorism clarified by Webster's definition of *art* as "skill derived from knowledge and experience."

## INFANCY

**Medical.** In large part, "mental hygiene" might well begin before the child is born. If the mother suffers dietary deficiencies during pregnancy, especially during the critical third to six month, or takes excessive doses of hormones, antibiotics, alcohol, or psychoactive drugs, or suffers severe emotional strains, the child she is carrying may be secondarily injured. Birth should, of course, be expertly conducted to prevent prolonged compression, and aftercare must ensure respiration, asepsis, and constant protection for the neonate, especially if it is premature.

**Early Metabolic Deficiencies.** On rare occasions, children are born with a congenital incapacity to metabolize galactose or other dietary elements such as the amino acid phenylalanine. Unless the deficiencies are detected within the first few weeks and special diets prescribed, these substances or their metabolic by-products accumulate and permanently injure the brain and other organs. Fortunately, reliable tests are now available for such hidden defects. There is no evidence that mother's milk is nutritionally superior to pediatric formulae, but if the infant is not breast-fed, it must in other ways be physically stimulated by rocking, fondling, and gentle play to promote its sensory and motor development and emotional responsiveness. Anna Freud, Margaret Mahler, and others have demonstrated that children given adequate physical care in orphanages but deprived of individualized love and attention during the crucial first four years of life lose the capacity for warm relationships and instead develop serious and persistent disturbances of behavior, variously called *protophrenia*, or *childhood schizophrenia*.

**Congenital Abnormalities.** The birth of a defective child may be due to an abnormal division of the fertilized ovum, or to neonatal or postnatal injuries, and is no certain indication of an "hereditary taint" in either parent. Maldeveloped extremities, cleft palate, or other deformaties are, of course, immediately apparent at birth, but it may take several weeks, months, or years to detect partial deafness, impaired vision, susceptibility to epileptic seizures, or mental and developmental retardation. Each child presents a highly individualized problem, but the general principles of procedure are these:

(a) If the infant is so seriously handicapped, either physically (e.g., without functional arms and legs) or mentally (I.Q. less than 50), that adequate adjustments outside a private or public insitution would be extremely difficult or impossible, then it may be to the child's and everyone else's advantage to arrange for prolonged hospitalization to develop its maximal potentials or to accept permanent institutional care. Parental rationalizations as to the "advantage of loving care at home until it outgrows its handicap" require a sympathetic hearing, but such pleas are usually based on threatened familial pride and attempts to deny reality rather than on objective considerations for the welfare of the handicapped child, its siblings, and its future associates.

(b) If the child's capacities permit extramural adaptations, its future happiness may be promoted as follows.

**Physical Handicaps.** Crossed eyes can be corrected by glasses, or by surgery before one eye becomes functionally useless. Congenitally malformed arms or legs can often be fitted with ingenious artificial prostheses that restore adequate function—an important consideration if the child is to have character-forming play and group experiences with peers who might otherwise reject and embitter him. By modern methods, even a deaf-mute can be taught to communicate, become literate, and perhaps develop unusual talents—as witness the classic example of Helen Keller.

**Intellectual Retardation.** Children with a reliable IQ rating below 75 should not be exposed to competition with other children at home or in standard schools, since they soon feel inferior and alienated. They may then regress to infantile helplessness, retreat into self-isolation, or develop patterns of rebellion and delinquency. Instead, they should first be given especially patient preparation at home, and then placed in classes for the "exceptional child," where their basic education and training in social skills can be paced more slowly and carefully. In rare but fortunate cases, special manual, linguistic, musical, or even mathematical potentials may be discovered and developed, which will compensate for defects in other spheres.

**Autism.** Characterized by bizarre movements, deviated attention span and blunted or distorted affects, autism is probably of genetic origin, requires prolonged medication and retraining, and may have a poor prognosis.

**Genetic Prospects.** It has been reliably estimated that over 85 percent of mental retardation in this country is nonhereditary, and that if every person with an intelligence quotient below 80 were prevented from having children, there would be no appreciable decrease of mental deficiency in future generations. Mental retardates therefore have every right to marry and have progeny unless, in special cases, a geneticist finds adequate reasons to the contrary.

**Precocity and Genius.** A different set of problems is presented by this opposite extreme. If a child's unusual intellectual, mechanical, artistic, or other capacities are not recognized early and given encouragement, expression, and approbation, he may become bored, frustrated, isolated, restless, contemptuous, and rebellious. Care must be taken, nevertheless, to keep his development physically and mentally rounded, else he too would miss the essentials of play and of peer and adult camaraderie that are indispensable to the development of social skills and allegiances.

## CHILDHOOD NEUROSES

Some children develop "perverse" feeding habits, "night terrors," bedwetting, school phobias, and other patterns of "problem behavior." In most cases, the child is reacting to familial insecurities arising from neglect, parental conflicts, excessive expectations, sibling rivalries, or other such threats to its essential dependencies. The child may also behave in ways to *invite* censure and physical "punishment"—not because it is "masochistic"—a paradoxical term (Chapter 5)—but because only in this manner can the child evoke concern and attention. If the parents refuse counselling for themselves, the therapist, by perceiving and temporarily fulfilling the child's needs, can partially substitute for delinquent parents, promote healthier peer and adult relationships, develop the child's skills and intellectual interests, and improve its social conduct despite adverse familial circumstances.

## PUBERTY

As indicated in chapter 8 pleasure in genital stimulation is present in both sexes almost from birth, and with the maturation of the sex glands genital drives become more intense. In many cultures the boys and girls are then initiated into ostensible adulthood through various puberty rites, even though they may be yet far from adequately prepared for mature responsibilities and still subject to many limitations and prohibitions, particularly in the sexual sphere. Libidinal urges may then find release in various ways. Among them:

**Displaced Eroticism** in exaggerated dress and hair styles, pornographic interests, sexually suggestive speech and mannerisms, pelvic-centered dancing to jejune musical tastes, and transient but intense "crushes" on erotized figures, with or without sexual adventures which may result in infections and pregnancies. Within the ranges of time, place, and culture, these may still be considered "normal" accompaniments of adolescent exuberance; however, excesses in any of them connote insecurity and escapism from underlying familial, educational, or social anxieties, and may indicate a need for empathetic counseling, environmental change, and redirection of interests.

## ADOLESCENCE

The years between puberty and the arbitrary ages of legal "adulthood" (E. Erikson), constitute an important period during which the adolescent must seek and acquire what he will call, often defiantly, his quasi-deified "Self." But in our almost incredibly intricate culture, with its multitudes of familial, educational, occupational, esthetic, economic, cultural, and other intertwined demands and relationships, the acquisition of an adequately multiadaptive yet unique individuality is an increasingly difficult task, even for the best prepared and talented of our youth; ergo, interim or permanent, partial or complete failures are to be expected. They may take the following forms singly or, much more frequently, in various combinations.

**Regressions** may occur to familial or other dependencies, as expressed in maladjustments at school, financial irresponsibilities, or minor delinquencies requiring repeated interventions and succorances by parents or guardians. These perennial "protectors" and "rescures" may protest loudly over the injustice of their fate, but are often secretly loath to give up vicarious gratifications in the adolescent's behavior—sometimes extended into his adulthood. Therapy must then include all affected members of the family constellation if their reciprocally neurotic relationships are to be dealt with and adverse consequences for all concerned prevented.

**Later Sterotypes.** If neither normal nor neurotic familial securities seem available or attractive, the adolescent or young adult may seek status in a peer group which permits a return to ostentatiously neglectful habits of hygiene, beards and tangled tresses, idiomatic modes of speech, outrageous dress and aesthetic tastes, hideouts in secreted shacks or "pads," exhibitionistic or deviated sexuality, and a pseudosophisticated lingo of avant-garde nihilism and social protest. Less escapist groupings are harmless or beneficial as interim experiences throughout youth—and indeed continue into normal adulthood in the form of cliques and societies with their prescribed uniforms, secret handclasps, passwords, rituals, and public professions of high social purpose, sometimes leading to actual public service. The dividing line is this: When an adolescent becomes so immersed in "extracurricular activities" as to neglect his education, physical health, and broader social development, or when he selects a group that advocates "sports" which endanger others (reckless drag racing), or promotes public obscenity, sexual arrogance, and gang violence, or indulges in escapes from reality through alcohol, "goof balls" (dexedrine), "red bullets" (seconal), "pot" (marijuana) or deleterious "psychedelic" drugs such as mescaline, lysergic acid, quaalude, cocaine, opiate derivatives or the more dangerous PCP ("angel dust"), or when he counters reasonable restraints with serious threats of vagrancy, delinquency or suicide,[2] then comprehensive therapy directed toward resolving physical, familial, and group insecurities, revealing newer opportunities and inculcating more practicable social loyalties and modes of conduct is urgently called for. This may, when necessary, be coordinated with famial, institutional, or even police discipline until healthy internal restraints and external adaptations are developed.

**Promiscuity.** The connotations of "promiscuity" vary widely even among Western cultures: In the Scandinavian lands, for example, teenagers in the upper social strata are expected to have lovers and mistresses; over 40 percent of pregnancies are conceived outside of marriage, and children born out of wedlock are raised by the State without onus of illegitimacy. In our own country, sexual customs are changing rapidly under pressure from our iconoclastic youth: formal "dating," often encouraged by upper middle-class parents, now frequently begins near puberty; "going steady" with a succession of 2- or 3-month partners is a status symbol in many a juvenile group and often involves "necking" or "petting" (including fondling of breasts and genitals) or "making out" to the extent of sexual intercourse. If and when these practices become even more widely and frankly accepted, the adolescent's fear of social reprisal will correspondingly diminish, but because of the inherent uncertainties and insecurities of this age period in our culture, the poignant rivalries, jealousies, disappointments, and reactive hostilities involved will require sympathetic hearings, interim reassurances, and active guidance toward more practicable and gratifying relationships.

**Identity Diffusion.** This term refers to another unfortunate eventuality: with so many competing demands and conflictual roles to play during high school and early college years, the late adolescent may spread himself thin trying to be simultaneously a brilliant scholar, a winning athlete, a popular leader, a cryptic mystic, a potent lover or seductive nymph, a cynical yet "involved" sophisticate, and a dozen other incompatible alteregos. The result is often a fragile superficiality in each role, and at worst, chaos and breakdown in all. As noted, this may be prevented by optimal collaboration between parents, teachers, and institutions in guiding each late adolescent in accordance with his limitations, motivations, and potentialities toward greater personal integrity and an adult career.

## SEXUAL AND MARITAL PROBLEMS

Many "living companionships" are being contracted by couples who, under the guise of undertaking mutual responsibilities, are really seeking dependent securities, extramarital sex, and rationalized escapes from legal obligations, parenthood, or other mature relationships. Under these circumstances, even if the couple eventually marries, disappointments and dissatisfactions are frequent and give rise to pervasive anxieties and depressions, sexual frigidity or impotence usually limited to the companion or spouse, and attempts at relief through drugs or alcohol, usually requiring both individual and joint therapy.

**The Role of Sex in Therapy.** It is a peculiar aspect of our present culture that in many circles a preoccupation with sexuality has become so fashionable that partners in a poorly planned and conducted liaison or marriage, after a few days to as many years of recurrent crises, will come to the therapist with the naive plea that if only their "sexual problems could be solved," their companionship could still somehow "be worked out." Accordingly, a specific request is often made for "instruction in sexual techniques," in the illusion that this will form a solid basis for compatibility.

The therapist can be aware that sexual diversions have always been sought by men and women as a temporary distraction from life's stresses, and have throughout history been expressed in pseudotherapeutic cults. One need but recall the aphrodisiac rites of Ishtar in Mesopotamia, the orgiastic Dionysian Mysteries of Greek and Roman times, and the open lasciviousness of later generations as celebrated by Petronius, Boccaccio, Rabelais, or Mailer. Today also, therapeutically rationalized[3] or cynically "sophisticated" erotic defiances and escapisms are sought in frenetic mate-combinations and permutations, not only by our restless youth, but also by the harassed executives and den mothers of split-level suburbia. Nevertheless, when a disillusioned supplicant insists that his or her difficulties, however avidly described, are "basically sexual," experienced therapists have learned also to explore the underlying insecurities, dependencies, frustrated ambitions, fears, hostilities, ambiguous values and social goals, or other spheres of conflict and uncertainty inadequately covered by Salome's seven veils of sexuality. When these more fundamental problems are solved through various forms of dynamic, comprehensive, reality-oriented dyadic or family therapy (not infrequently the group may have to include self-seeking extramarital "love partners," interfering "friends" and in-laws, or even contentious attorneys), the sexual difficulties, which are usually secondary defensive, escapist, or compensatory epiphe-

nomena, disappear in most instances with predictable and gratifying regularity (Chapter 15, Cases 3, 4, 5).

## THERAPY IN THE MIDDLE YEARS

Mild anxiety states, minor reactive depressions, and accompanying psychosomatic dysfunctions may first be relieved by
medication, both for its specific and placebo (L., I please you) effects, as indicated in Chapter 12. With rapport thus enhanced,
tactful, perceptive inquiry will nearly always elicit an illuminating account of the patient's anxieties, doubts, fears, and per-
plexities, accompanied by appeals for sympathy, advice, and,
not infrequently, personal service sometimes extending beyond
strict professional limits (Chapters 5 and 6). Perceptive empathy rather than sympathy (which some patients take to mean
they have, after all, always been "right" and the world always
"wrong") may be expressed; however, indulgent partisanships
and personal interferences should be avoided as generally leading to complications for all concerned, and guidance given only
in the sense of helping patients reorder their lives according to a
simple truism: *improve what can yet be changed and make the best of
the rest*, to wit:

**Reorientation.** Rut-formed patterns can gradually be altered
to possible advantage: goals modified, old interests and friendships renewed, fresh ones cultivated, and broader horizons of
life explored. Care must be taken, however, to conserve what is
still valuable in the patient's life: only occasionally will a defiant
resignation, an impulsive move to a strange environment, a late
shuffling of marital partners, or other such major changes solve
more problems than they evoke.

**Adaptation.** Readjustments must be made in accordance
with another ancient aphorism: happiness is not a simple sum-
mation of material or interpersonal acquisitions or guarantees,
but the *ratio between what is possessed and what is desired*. In effect, if
the patient will scale down his demands to approximately what is

available, contentment is obviously within reach. One set of tennis doubles or a leisurely nine holes of golf may be enjoyed almost as thoroughly as three sets of tennis singles, waterskiing, or ice-boating used to be. Sexual intercourse once every week or two may furnish more satisfying orgasms than partial impotence or long-delayed ejaculations experienced in more frequent attempts at coitus. The position of accountant, shop foreman, rewrite man, or associate professor may, on rational reflection, be considered as more secure and comfortable than those of chief auditor, company president, city editor or departmental chairman. Interpersonally, the devotion of spouse, children, and grandchildren can still be earned rather than demanded, provided control and exploitation are no longer considered one's due. These reevaluations may at first be rejected by the patient as an unconscionable surrender of his cherished and capitalized "Self-Image," but careful and repeated reviews of alternatives usually lead to more realistic physical and social expectations on the patient's part and correspondingly more rational behavior.

## THE CLIMACTERIUM

The disorders of mood and conduct that occur in some "middle"- or "upper-class" women during their fifth decade of life may still be attributed by them to the physical effects of the menopause, so that they can conveniently blame their erratic and troubled behavior on a metabolic imbalance beyond their control. Indeed, so avidly do some cling to this rationalization that they will go from one physician to another demanding medicine or injections of vitamins and hormones (or to nonmedical practitioners for diets, baths, massages, exercises, or covert sex) intended to deny or reverse the dreaded "change of life." True, minute quantities of estrogens and progesterones administered in proper sequence may help relieve the "hot flashes" and "dizzy spells" (vasomotor disturbances), transient palpitations, and mild abdominal and muscular cramps that sometimes occur during the cessation of ovulation, but this does little to resolve concurrent psychologic problems.

So also, it has become fashionable for some men, especially

those in higher economic echelons, to blame their difficulties on a parallel "male climacterium" and to demand therapy with pituitary or testicular extracts. However, the difficulties experienced by both sexes in later middle age—which, in the larger sense of wrenching reorientations as to accomplishments to date, current liabilities versus assets and anticipations of the future, do indeed necessitate a sometimes poignantly painful "change of life"—may be summarized as follows:

**Female.** On the physical side, feminine verve, beauty, and sexual attractiveness undeniably fade despite all artificial aids, and can no longer command flattering attentions from husbands and other men whose interests unmistakably begin to wander elsewhere. Divorces may occur, social successes diminish, old friends become self-preoccupied, and younger, more energetic women are elected to the Chairmanship of Hadassah, the district PTA, or the annual Charity Bazaar. Worse, sons and daughters grow up, depart for school and careers, marry, and ever more frankly and firmly resent attempts at continued maternal control. All that seems to remain is a life with less and less adventure, achievement, influence, or satisfactions—a dour and depressing vista. If renewed social climbing, frenetic extramarital flirtations, martyred protests about the ingratitude of husband, children, and friends, or increasing doses of tranquilizers all prove ineffective, one recourse remains: blame the recurrent anxieties and episodes of restless melancholy on failing glands rather than failing adaptabilities, and demand that the therapist—usually a physician required to act simultaneously as internist, gynecologist, father confessor, wailing wall, counselor, platonic lover, and magician—reverse time, restore past graces and glories, and prevent inexorable senescence (Chapter 15, Case 10).

**Male.** In their forties or fifties many men in our culture must also undergo, to use a hackneyed but appropriate phrase, quite agonizing reappraisals of their past, present and future. Advancing decrepitude of physique becomes undeniable, and sexual prowess—equated by many with general strength and virility—also begins to fail under the demands of increasingly frantic testing.[4] Occupational and social limitations must likewise be faced: unrealistic ambitions must be given up and efforts bent to the humiliating task of retaining one's present position against younger, better prepared competitors. Friends on whom one relied for help may have escalated out of reach or are faring worse than oneself—and in the latter case become awkward liabilities. The wife and children have become disillusioned and either complain openly of their familial disappointments or assume a martyred, maddeningly patronizing air toward "poor Dad, who meant well, so we'll try not to say anything to hurt his feelings." In short, life has, not fulfilled the confident expectations of youth and early manhood—and ahead lies nothing but increasingly bleak and lonesome old age. Perhaps—just perhaps —all this can still be changed by the concentrated vigor contained in the proper vitamin or hormone pill, or a dose of renewed masculinity injected through a syringe; ergo, the aging gladiator fervently hopes that some physician—or goat gland engrafter, naturopath, chiropractor, or other necromancer— can cure the temporary gonadal imbalance involved. If that is not the case, then some Hubbardian "scientologist," Buchmanite faith healer, Christian Scientist, or T-group leader can Clear his Conscious, Disipate his Suppressed Complexes, Correct his Errors of Thought, Release a Primal Scream, Utilize Latent Sensitivities and Potencies, and so bring about a Physical Rebirth or a Superconscious Enlightenment that will dispel the gathering doubts and shadows. But faith does not always spring eternal to counter melancholy; and rage, depression, and disorganization may ensue. Therapy must therefore proceed with the special empathy, tact, wisdom, and opportunism previously outlined (Chapter 15, Case 13).

## PROBLEMS OF AGING

**Ethology and Ethnology.** Our animal cousins, like ourselves, treat their aged according to the needs of differing social orders. Ruminants such as the red deer cherish and protect elderly cows and bucks, since experienced survivors can lead the herd to remote trails and pasturages unknown to the young. In contrast, predatory wolves exile their aged to fend for themselves after they can no longer participate in and earn their share of the pack's kill. In human parallels, good gray Hippocrates was revered in Hellenic times as a wise philosopher and physician, and in republican Rome the seniors of the city governed in the Senate. So, also, in the peaceful and esthetic Finnish Golden Era (as idealized in the Kalevala), the elderly were romantically cherished because they knew the songs and sagas that recounted the glory of their ancient race. In stark contrast, if the communal food supply became insufficient among the Labrador Eskimos during a hard winter, the patriarch was expected to leave the village and quietly freeze to death—yet, since the eldest son accompanied him part way on this journey to bid him farewell, the oldster felt that he was still revered and would, therefore, in a wishful fantasy immanent in all of us (see Oedipus at Colonus, chapter 2) be rewarded in some more pleasant land beyond.

In our culture the progressive disabilities of the senium (i.e., diminished capacity to perceive, categorize, differentiate, evaluate the environment, and to respond in a properly contingent and efficient fashion), the *reactions* of the aging individual significantly color his attempts to compensate for failing powers and threatened status by corresponding intensification of basic Ur- defenses. Physically, the presenile tries strenuously to reassert his waning vigor in various activities, from gardening through golf to gynecophilia; socially, to preempt whatever human relationships remain available to him; and to adopt and avidly defend philosophic or religious systems that deny death and promise some form of immortality.

Although a reasonable tolerance for disappointments and social neglect is a recourse to be acquired long before the senium, one should, while still young, develop a variety of interests, activities, and satisfactions that can be continued throughout life. Literature, music, art, philosophy—these are perennial joys, and almost independent of retained skills. He who loves the seas and still knows the proper rig and trim of a ship invites the respect and company of sailors of all ages.

**Therapy.** The first consideration is to grant our elders beliefs and practices that we ourselves will eventually cherish. If dear old Uncle Harry preaches that yoga or yogurt will make him a centenarian, or if aging Aunt Harriet believes that she still looks enticing in a revealing dress, such foibles up to the point of inviting social derision may be charitably condoned as relatively harmless. With regard to avidity for cants and cults, great men in their last years professed some fairly odd philosophies: the sociologist Auguste Comte literally worshipped his dead wife Clothilde as Queen of a Heavenly Society; the cosmologist Arthur Eddington considered God but a fellow-mathematician; Sir Oliver Lodge became an ardent Spiritualist; and Sigmund Freud himself, facing his fatal cancer, symbolically mastered it by including an "instinct for death" (*Thanatos*) in his metapsychology.

However, maintained social contacts and controls are also necessary. If these are not furnished along constructive channels, the aged may retreat to querulous dependencies and in a sense demand indulgent baby-sitters for their second childhood. In contrast, if they are given continued opportunities to exercise their remaining occupational and social skills, the cycle of familial disruption and parasitism may be long postponed (Chapter 15, Case 15).

As may be inferred, the therapy of the elderly is, whenever possible, best conducted where they can retain, at least in part, their status as senior citizens still valued by their community. Indeed, this attitude applies also in the unique filial *transference-countertransference relationships*, in that many aged like to picture the therapist or social worker not as an authoritative person, but as a dutiful son or daughter properly devoted to the oldster's interests. Such members of a family do not question, let alone imprison, their elders; instead, they visit with them, discuss mutual concerns respectfully and are rewarded by advice and benedictions—hence the many advantages of tactfully arranged home care plans as alternatives to even the most aseptic and "best conducted Hospices for the Incurable Aged."

**Institutional.** However, if hospitalization becomes necessary, the objectives must be changed from total custody to provisions for relieving the family and the community of the most burdensome aspects of caring for their aged member continuously. The family can be assured that during episodes of illness, or even if they simply want a vacation, they will have some place to leave the elderly member. This relief can range from 2 or 3 hours a day, through a day or two a week, to continuous inpatient residence for several months—but rarely with the intent of "terminal commitment." By this means the community's conscience is neither overstrained nor lulled, whereas the family, under this combined surveillance and succorance, resumes its lightened but remaining obligations.

**Therapy of the Dying.**If the patient has had a fulfilling life of affection and creativity,[5] and if the hygiene of the later years outlined above has been followed, the dying patient will approach the inevitable more like a Socrates than a Beethoven. The terminal days should be as free of physical pain as drugs, including marijuana, cocaine or opiates, can make them; as free of social isolation as family and friends can provide; and as serene about memories of past rewards and/or anticipation of those deserved in an afterlife as philosophers or clerics can imply or promise. Near death, as in life, man still longs for the Ur-comforts of physical ease, interpersonal empathy, and mystic transcendence that have been the themes of this volume—and deserves their fulfillment as each of us will in our time of undeniable bodily extinction.

## NOTES

1. Recent insurance proposals for fixed fees for the therapy of patients relegated to stereotyped "diagnostic related groups" (DRGs)

2. Such threats may not be idle: suicide rates have doubled among adolescents in the last 15 years (P.C. Holinger).

3. An intriguing example of what might be called erototherapy was the Celestial Bed in Dr. James Graham's Temple of Health in London, an "Institution Dedicated to the Cure of all Diseases," and thus advertised to both sexes in the Madison Avenue panegyrics of sevenscore years ago: "The Grand Celestial

Bed, whose medical influences are now celebrated from Pole to Pole and from the Rising to the Setting of the Sun, is twelve feet long by nine feet wide, supported by Forty Pillars of brilliant glass of the most exquisite workmanship in richly variegated colors.

"On the uppermost summit of the dome are placed two exquisite figures of Cupid (Eros) and Psyche, with a figure of Hymen behind . . . supporting a Celestial Crown sparkling over a pair of great loving turtle-doves on a little bed of roses. . . . At the head of the bed appears, sparkling with electrical fire, the Great First [sic] Commandment: 'Be fruitful, multiply and replenish the earth!'"

This enticing notice went on to imply that suitable partners would also be furnished as required—thus anticipating the use of "expert surrogates" in the therapy of impotence in males or frigidity in women, as recently also advocated by Masters and Johnson and other sex therapists.

4.  One of my patients defined anxiety as "the first time one cannot perform twice in one night," and panic as "the second time one cannot once."

5.  For masterpieces in science, literature, philosophy, art and music bequeathed to humanity by geniuses aged 65 and over, see H. Lehman, W. Dennis and E. Menkowski.

# Chapter 15

# CLINICAL ILLUSTRATIONS

The following necessarily limited[1] selection of 16 patient vignettes can only tangentially indicate the almost infinite variations, combinations, and permutations of human responses to stress. Each "case" has been given a stereotyped DSM III (Appendix I) code number to indicate what is now required for "diagnostic related group" (DRG) hospital compensation; however, as emphasized throughout this volume, every patient also presents various intensities of anxiety, obsessive-compulsive preoccupations, somatic dysfunctions, and covert and overt sociopathic, paranoid, or schizoid reactions which significantly modify prognosis and therapy (Chapter 4).

All names and other data in these case illustrations are clinically significant, but have no reference to any persons living or dead.

## ROSTER OF CASE ILLUSTRATIONS

**Case**

1. The Penurious Man
2. Somatization Disorder

3. Obsessive-Compulsive Disorder
4. Atypical Somatoform Disorder
5. Counterphobic Reaction
6. Anxiety-phobic Reaction
7. Sociopathic Personality; Criminality
8. Conversion Neurosis; Military
9. Atypical Impulse Control; Alcoholic Delirium
10. Midlife Adjustment Disorder
11. Schizophrenia with Symbolic Dereism
12. Psychophysiologic Dysfunctions; Schizophrenia
13. Hypomania
14. Psychogenic Pain Disorder
15. Geriatric Personality Disorder
16. Family Therapy; Forensic Aspects

## CASE 1: THE PENURIOUS MAN (301.84)

For an historical perspective, herewith a description of "an obsessive-compulsive personality" written two and a half millenia ago by Theophrastus, Aristotle's successor at the Academy of Athens.

"A Penurious Man is one who goes to a debtor to ask for his half-obol interest before the end of the month. At a dinner where expenses are shared he counts the number of cups each person drinks, and he makes a smaller libation to Artemis than anyone. When his servant breaks a pot or a plate, he deducts the value from his food. If his wife drops a copper, he moves furniture, beds, chests, and hunts in the curtains . . . He forbids anyone to pick a fig in his garden, to walk on his land, to pick up an olive or a date. Every day he goes to see that the boundary marks of his property have not been moved. He will dun a debtor and exact compound interest . . . He forbids his wife to lend anything —neither salt nor lamp-wick nor cinnamon nor marjoram nor meals nor garlands nor cakes for sacrifices. "All these trifles", he says, "mount up in a year." To sum up, the coffers of penurious men are moldy and the keys rust; they wear cloaks which hardly reach the thigh; a very little oil-bottle supplies them for anointing; they have hair cut short and do not put on their shoes until midday; and when they take their cloak to the fuller they urge him to use plenty of earth so that it will not be spotted so soon." It is evident that in this interesting literary portrait Theophrastus skillfully elaborates the various expressions of a single "personality trait"—penuriousness—and, indeed, describes behavior patterns recognizable in certain guardians of academic and research purse-strings today. It is equally obvious, however, that in order to preserve this simple unidimensional approach, Theophrastus makes no attempt to canvass the total character of the "penurious man:" his taste in music, his bravery in battle, his religious beliefs, his skill and delight in throwing a javelin, or his devotion to his country or his children (Chapter 4).

### CASE 2: SOMATIZATION DISORDER AMAUROSIS (300.81)

A fifteen year-old girl with intense sexual curiosity contrived to witness parental intercourse. However, when she was discovered and chastised she suffered an attack of "blindness" which greatly troubled her parents. Symptomatically effective therapy consisted of an ophthalmoscopic examination, a few face-saving drops of saline into her eyes, avuncular explanations to the patient about the eventually counterproductive effects of her behaviors and advice to the parents to discourage further adolescent historionics by benign neglect.

### CASE 3: OBSESSIVE-COMPULSIVE DISORDER; FAMILIAL AND RELIGIOUS (300.30)

A twenty-year-old wife was referred by her internist for compulsive mouth washing, sexual frigidity, and episodes of nausea and vomiting which were especially severe on weekends. After rapport was established, she hesitantly associated her symptoms to fellatio with her new husband. This revulsion was symbolically exacerbated on Sundays when, as a devout Catholic, she swallowed the sacramental wafer symbolizing Christ's body, which she fantasied as "also His penis." The first concern was mitigated by assurances as to the normal range of marital techniques; the second was resolved with the aid of an empathetic and benevolent priest, who explained that the cloths that traditionally cover Christ's pubic region in religious art are there to conceal from profane eyes his ethereal and angelic asexuality. With further marital counseling as to related conflicts over precoital sex play, contraception, in-law intrusions, and other familial tensions, the patient's concerns abated, and the placebos that had been substituted for her previous medications were discontinued.

### CASE 4: ATYPICAL SOMATOFORM DISORDER (300.71) WITH MARITAL THERAPY

A twenty-two-year-old married woman, of normal intelligence but limited educational background, was referred by an obstetrician because, for a year after the delivery of a stillborn baby complicated by a mild puerperal thrombophlebitis she had continued to have an inexplicable spastic paralysis of her right leg.

**Anamnesis** At the age of eighteen she had married an illiterate, stolid, but devoted suitor, mainly because she desired to escape from the drudgery of factory work; however, she had instead been obliged to assume the unexpected responsibilities of a wife and mother. Her first child, delivered with difficulty, was born deformed, and its care added greatly to her burdens and disillusionments. Within a few months, she was pregnant again, and this time she had an even more stormy pregnancy, terminated by stillbirth and a residual thrombophlebitis. In treatment for the latter complications, the obstetrician prescribed rest, warm packs, light massage, and—psychologically most important to the patient—a suspension of intercourse until she was "completely recovered." The husband remained continent for months, but his growing impatience forced the patient again to seek treatment for what she called, with significant lack of anxiety, her "chronic milk leg."[2] In the psychiatric interview the patient naively stated that her leg "was better all day," yet so painfully stiff in adduction at night that intercourse with her husband was impossible. However, the patient soon recognized the symptom's relationship to her fears of a third pregnancy, although her self-respect and rapport were preserved by never making this point traumatizingly explicit. The therapy was then implemented by inducing her husband, through appeals to his own needs, to retain his wife's affection by practicing Catholic contraceptive techniques they both would accept: after this the patient, her leg, and her husband were reunited in various marital functions.

### CASE 5: COUNTERPHOBIC REACTION (300.0)

A young woman came bearing a sealed note from her internist which read: "Miss . . . has a blood pressure of 240/142 and has probably been severely hypertensive for at least 2 years, but she says she has had no symptoms at all. Next week she's to have an abdomina sympathectomy and she knows it's a fairly dangerous operation with probably a long and uncomfortable convalescence. But that doesn't seem to faze her either. Is she schizophrenic or really suicidal?"

True enough, when the patient—a winsomely attractive girl—was interviewed, she stated at first that, apart from occasional slight headaches, she "felt fine" and if the doctors thought she needed a serious operation, "the thing to do was to have it and not worry about it." Far from schizoid, however, was her sympathetic interest in everything and everyone about her, her facile responses to all topics under discussion other than her own illness, and the friendly rapport she cultivated.

Briefly, her psychiatric history revealed that her parents were cultured, artistic people devoted to their only daughter, that her home life had been relatively happy, and that she had been popular and successful at school and college—far more because of her ingratiating good humor and extraverted activities than her outstanding scholastic abilities. Early in life she had become interested in dramatics, had cultivated her voice under expert tutelage, and had starred in high school and college productions. A talent scout had witnessed her performance in one of these and had offered her a contract for a role in a traveling operetta company. The patient had been overjoyed, since she considered this a start on a long-coveted stage career. Correspondingly great, therefore, was her disappointment when a routine physical examination for participation in Actors' Equity insurance revealed a degree of vascular hypertension which made a stage career impracticable. The patient's reactions were characteristic: she denied the seriousness of her illness to herself as well as to others, trustingly put herself into the hands of her physicians, and blithely planned to fulfill her contract after the "slight delay" of her operation. However, those defensive denials were gradually breached in sympathetic interviews until the patient confided that she had really been suffering from headaches, tinnitus, vertigo, fatigue, and other symptoms for several years, had wished to seek help, but had feared to do so because a serious disorder might be diagnosed. Finally, she confessed, with what was an unconvincing attempt at nonchalance, that if she could not continue her dramatic career, she would hardly consider life really worth living and suicide would be the only solution.

Under therapy, she was able to change her dysthymia from a brittle pretense of unconcern to a more confident and stable courage, after which a sympathectomy was performed. She cooperated well during convalescence and left the hospital relieved of her hypertension by the operation and by diazide medication. With analytic guidance, she also developed a relatively realistic acceptance of her physical limitations and made alternative plans for interim support by her well-to-do family until an equally creative and satisfying career as a playwright could be attained.

### CASE 6: ANXIETY-PHOBIC DISORDER (300.30) WITH HOMICIDAL PANIC (300.01)

A twenty-two-year-old laborer complained of attacks of palpitation and faintness that had begun 2 months previously, and which he attributed to "heart disease from overwork." The history revealed that he had been raised in privation in the slums of a steel town, had received relatively little formal education, and had grown up with strong resentments against an economic system that, he felt, sentenced him to a life of squalor and drudgery. His hostilities had been intensified by exhausting work in a steel mill until, seeking group support, he joined a radical organization pledged to a program of violent revolution. His assignment was to advance himself in the mill until he "could strike from inside." Because of his skill and intelligence, he was rapidly promoted to a well-paid and responsible job: operating a huge crane that transferred iron ore from a lake freighter to an open-hearth furnace. The patient gloried in his work so long as an instructor was with him to prevent any mistakes in operation. However, the first day he was trusted alone in the control turret he began to experience severe anxiety that soon centered about a single obsessional impulse; namely, that with one pull of a lever he could so manipulate his gargantuan machine as to wreck the dock, sink the ship and probably kill several men. As he pictured this his heart pounded, his hand trembled, his vision blurred, and his knees grew weak; finally these and other subjective and physiologic manifestations grew so severe that he applied for sick leave and to the University Clinic for therapy.

This consisted of rest, mild sedation, and a thorough examination conducted so that complete reports as to the patient's physical competence could be sent to his employers. With sympathetic understanding and guidance, the patient—an intelligent and essentially honest individual—recognized that his anxieties and obsessions had their origin in conflicts between his lifelong hostilities as recently opposed by occupational loyalties. As insight developed and new securities in therapeutic and group relationships were formed, his anxieties and concomitant symptoms fairly rapidly abated. Fortunately, too, his aggressions were further disarmed when the company he had worked for proved entirely cooperative in paying his hospital fees, giving him an interim vacation, and then offering him a choice of several other jobs. The patient returned to work, found his new duties almost entirely to his liking, and remained symptom-free.

## CASE 7: SOCIOPATHIC PERSONALITY DISORDER
## (301.89); PROGRESS TO CRIMINALITY

Toni was the second of nine siblings, and was scarcely a year old before his mother had to shift her remaining minimal attention to another newborn sister. At the age of four Toni was toddling the streets unattended; at twelve he and his elder brother were already members of a semi-delinquent street gang. With little security and less guidance at home, Toni quickly adopted the code of his successful gang leaders: "right" meant obedience, safety, and advancement; "smart" to steal, lie, be "tough" and to live for one's immediate gain; *stupido* was to be unsuccessful; "chicken," to submit to parental, educational, police or other unnecessary discipline.

For Toni, then, most teachers and all policemen were to be outwitted. In his short schooling he was as truant as it was safe to be, and in jobs after school he stole within an accurately judged probability of discovery. Equipped with native cunning, courage, and charisma, he soon became the leader of a local Mafiaesque "family" for organized crime. This rise was encouraged by his father, who profited indirectly by the boy's increasing earnings and local status; indeed, the father began to use what political influence he had to get the lad special considerations from the local police, while the mother remained almost totally ignorant of the direction of her son's development. Other influences on the boy's life were few and deceptive. Toni took a liking to the parish priest and not only kept his church immune from vandalism, but even sang in the choir—thereby convincing the priest of the lad's inherent purity of soul. Similarly, there were other "right guys" in the neighborhood, among them compliant saloon keepers and minor politicians who, on Toni's orders, were protected from local depredations, thus adding to Toni's allies in sometimes influential quarters.

Toni progressed from petty embezzlements on newspaper collections to acting as a fence for stolen tires, to bootlegging and finally to "protection" of graft and gambling. Sexually, he was arrogant and promiscuous—and yet by his own lights strictly moral: his friends' sisters or fiancees were rebuffed when they attempted to seduce him. He remained loyal to his ethnic group, generous to his parents, siblings and friends, and indefatigable in working for any sentimental cause that, however unpredictably, appealed to him. Yet when he thought it profitable he could also arrange to have a local businessman who had offended him ruined by intimidation or actual destruction of property, or with righteous equanimity order a member of his gang beaten severely for some neglect or error.

Eventually, when he demanded blackmail from a politician too highly placed, he was arrested and could barely manage to be tried by a judge who, though properly bribed, could do no more than give him a choice "as a first offender" between jail or enlisting in the Army "to learn to be a good citizen." Toni, sure he could "beat the rap" anywhere, duly applied, but when, on the basis of his recent police record and a discerning psychiatric examination, he was rejected, his pride was deeply wounded. He therefore secured certification from a local physician as to his physical health, obtained "character references" from his parish priest and several local businessmen, and so armed, reappealed for induction.

The appeal panel then faced this problem: Toni hated authority and there was every indication that once his pride had been assuaged by induction, he would be as chronic a troublemaker in the Army as he had been in civil life. He might eventually place himself at the head of a group of likespirited rebels to disrupt routine and discipline and even endanger their outfit in combat. Before the panel could reach an agreement their problem was solved: in the interim an overconfident Toni had also challenged the authentic branch of the Chicago Mafia—with fatal pretherapeutic results.

### CASE 8: CONVERSION NEUROSIS (300.11); MILITARY IMPLICATIONS

A twenty-eight-year-old man complained that since his recent service in the Navy he had suffered from episodes of "a stifling in my chest and a feeling of being all tensed up and in a cold sweat. I wanted to run away from I wouldn't know what." These symptoms almost invariably occurred when he heard a loud, unexpected noise, when he was forced to ride in a crowded conveyance, or when he had to wait his turn in a line of people. He had built up various protective patterns such as avoiding crowds, walking up stairs instead of taking elevators, and insisting on absolute quiet at home or wearing cotton in his ears, but his "waking spells" had continued to be frequent and severe and his sleep increasingly disturbed by a repetitive dream in which he tried desperately to reach the head of a column of people, always failed, and then woke in a state of deep apprehension.

*Physical and laboratory findings* were normal except for a high basal metabolic rate.

**Anamnesis.** The patient had led a somewhat sheltered life, but had made consistent educational and vocational progress and had become a trusted executive in an insurance firm. He had married happily, and had shown no overt neurotic symptoms until the onset of his presenting complaints.

**Present Illness.** After several interviews (one under light Amytal hypnosis), the patient began to trace many of his difficulties to his experiences during naval training. At first, he recalled only self-defensive "screen memories" in which the Navy, and not he, was made to appear at fault. As an "economically minded citizen" he had been "outraged" by what he saw of Navy practice, such as reckless waste of food, tossing soiled dishes or blankets overboard instead of washing them, and extravagant purchases of useless items. Gradually, however, as his personal guilts became more evident and his anxieties over them more acceptable, the following memories emerged.

He had held up fairly well during the often irrational routines of boot training, until sent to sea and assigned to a team in the magazine deck of a destroyer, where he was trained to pass ammunition through a mechanical elevator to the gun crews above. He experienced considerable fear on initial contact with the imminent dangers involved, and was always the first to take his place in line at drills for "evacuate post" or "abandon ship."

However, he was able to find two sources of security: the generally high morale of the ship and a feeling of personal pride in the smooth efficiency of his ammunition squad. One day, however, one of the most skillful members of his team dropped a live shell on the deck—a harmless occurrence in itself, but one that represented to the patient the possibility of a magazine explosion that would mean certain death. The next day he noted a peculiar stiffness in his right arm and shoulder that interfered increasingly with his work of lifting shells from a rack to the elevator. The medical officer, noting the muscular tension and the limitations of joint motion, suspected arthritis and sent the patient to sick bay. Here, 2 days later, the patient heard that an explosion in the magazine of another ship had indeed killed eight men. Anxiety attacks grew intense and frequent, his nights increasingly sleepless, and he became so susceptible to startle reactions in response to sudden noises or flashes of light that the functional nature of his illness was recognized. Unfortunately, no therapy was instituted, and the patient was given a medical discharge. He returned home, where his arm rapidly improved; nevertheless, his anxiety attacks and his associated fears of crowds, elevators, and naval scenes continued unabated. One other episode illustrated the semantic spread of these symbolisms: when he returned to work, his employer welcomed him, but explained that since his old associates had been promoted during the interim expansion of the company, the patient "would have to take his place in line" for his turn at advancement. Although this was expected, the phrase "place in line" itself induced a severe attack of anxiety and uncontrolled sobbing. Subsequent episodes of emotional instability characterized by cardiac palpitations, faintness, and other somatic manifestations eventually led to his hospitalization.

**Therapy.** In brief, this consisted of initial sedation to control insomina and general tension, and a complete diagnostic checkup to allay the patient's half-wishful "fears" that he was suffering from some serious physical disease instead of a humiliating "nervous breakdown." When adequate rapport had been gained, his symbolic defenses against latent anxiety were traced to his military experiences, and preliminary "intellectual" insight was thus established. Concurrently, he was reintroduced into previously avoided activities: a ride on the hospital elevator first with the therapist, then a nurse, and finally alone, passage through a noisy basement preparatory to participating in team bowling, and eventually, viewing a movie on naval gunnery. Incidental marital and occupational conflicts were concurrently also resolved in dyadic and family conferences, and the patient returned to work relatively symptom-free 3 weeks after admission for only occasional outpatient follow-up.

### CASE 9: ATYPICAL IMPULSE CONTROL DISORDER (312.39) WITH ALCOHOLIC DELIRIUM (292.81) AND DYSTHYMIA (300.40)

A twenty-seven-year-old patient was admitted to the university hospital in acute alcoholic delirium: disorientated, ridden by fearful hallucinations, and confusedly amnestic. After 2 days of rest, mild sedation, hydrotherapy, and high caloric feeding, he was able to give this account of his life experiences.

**Anamnesis.** At an early age he had suffered from acute rheumatic fever which left him with painful joints and impaired cardiac function. His father—a self-reliant and highly religious but apparently ignorant and unfeeling man—had then taken a strong dislike to his "weakling" son and had made numerous compensatory demands on him, including almost impossibly high requirements as to his scholastic performance. Despite the additional necessity for partial self-support, the patient completed junior college and undertook special training for an accountant's certificate. The strain, however, impaired his health, and at the age of twenty-one he had to be admitted to a municipal sanatorium for apical tuberculosis. He took even this with good grace, cooperated well in his treatment, and was making progress toward recovery when he became enamored of a girl who was about to leave the sanatorium. Understandably fearful of losing her, the patient persuaded the hospital physician—who apparently let his romantic paternalism affect his medical judgment—to sign a premature discharge, and the couple were married soon afterward.

Misfortunes, however, promptly begin to pile up at a rate that would hardly be given credence outside the Book of Job. The patient's wife, dissatisfied with his salary as a bank clerk, insisted that he resume his study for a CPA examination, and in his devotion to her he again taxed his strength and resistance dangerously. A defalcation was next discovered in the bank's accounts, and for several harrowing weeks the patient was under unjust suspicion. While he was suspended and under technical bail, his wife left him with no explanation other than a note to the effect that she "couldn't any longer tolerate a physical weakling, and especially a thief." Two days later, the patient was completely cleared of all responsibility in the bank theft, only to be told by the bank manager who had originally accused him, that "for obvious reasons, we can no longer work together" and that the patient would therefore have to resign his position. That night, in a fit of coughing, the patient for the first time in months brought up blood-streaked sputum—a strong indication that his tuberculosis was reactivated, and quite probably more seriously than ever. With everything gone: job, wife, and even marginal health, the patient bribed a druggist—the first illegal act in his life—and secured a bottle of barbiturates for a planned suicide. However, he also reached a preliminary decision: since sober habits, hard study, honest work, and marital devotion had brought nothing but frustration, illness, and sorrow, before he died he was going to have an orgy, however brief, of defiant self-indulgence. Not knowing quite how to go about this, he collected all his available funds and began with what he had heard the men at his office boast of: he went to a locally notorious tavern, picked out one of the most expensive "hostesses," and set out on his lethal celebration. Presumably unaware of his purpose but receptive of his method, she bought a plentiful supply of liquor with his money, accompanied him home, and there continued to ply him with drink until he was in a confused stupor, after which she appropriated a considerable fee for her services and left him to his own devices. The next day the patient was found in a state of active delirium by a neighbor who had previously liked the patient as an unobtrusive, friendly person, and who now rightly reasoned that he "must be out of his mind to act this way." Fortunatley, the neighbor refrained from calling a police ambulance and instead brought the patient to the university hospital for medical care.

**Therapy.** This was first directed to meet the patient's urgent physiologic needs (Ur I) and then toward his social rehabilitation (Ur II). After the initial therapy outlined above, the pulmonary tuberculosis was surgically controlled by a partial pneumothorax, and the rheumatic valve lesion was compensated by cardiac medication. The bank manager was summoned for an interview and, as was to be expected, came in a patronizing "I-knew-he-was-odd all-the-time" attitude. However, when an appeal was made to his "humanitarian sympathies" supplemented by an implied concern that if the patient remained embittered he might take legal action against the bank, the manager, with a newly harried air of "let bygones be bygones," decided to reemploy the patient at an increased salary. Next, the patient's wife was interviewed, and her own fears of friendless ill-health and her needs for security and alleviation of guilt were utilized to effect a reconciliation with the patient. With his most pressing problems thus partially resolved, the patient was discharged from the hospital, but with arrangements for interviews at weekly intervals to help guide the couple through their initial readjustments. When seen in a final individual session 6 months later, he reported that he had passed his accountancy examinations, had been promoted to the position of chief teller at his bank, was fairly happy in his work and in his marriage, and had experienced no further serious difficulties.

### CASE 10: MIDLIFE ADJUSTMENT DISORDER (309.40), RAPPORT REORIENTATION AND RESOCIALIZATION

A forty-five-year-old socially prominent woman was referred for episodes of severe anxiety and depression, excessive intake of alcohol and tranquilizers, and intimations of suicide.

Apparently conforming to her experiences with several previous therapists, she immediately launched a mélange of devastating criticisms of her parents, siblings, friends, and former therapists, embroidered with fanciful childhood recollections, dream interpretations, and other such pseudoanalytic persiflage. To avoid encouraging these evasive tactics, the therapist made almost no comments until her fourth session. On that occasion she came in limping and, on inquiry, replied that she had stepped on the prongs of a rake in her rose garden that morning. She then again plunged into gratuitious "interpretations" to the effect that this obviously signified her youthful relations with "an introjected brother" who had been considered a "sexually promiscuous rake;" that, when the rake handle rose up, it symbolized his penile erection; that the bleeding from her foot signified both her defloration and an incestuous abortion; and so on with similarly fantastic "free association." When this subtly derisive litany was finally interrupted by the therapist's request that he examine her injured foot, she professed to be shocked by his manifest "voyeurism"—and then considered herself symbolically "impregnated" when he tested and then administered tetanus toxoid gluteally to counter the dangers presented by an obviously dirt-contaminated wound.

Nevertheless, this incident dramatically changed the whole course of her treatment. Reassured by the evidence of the therapist's realistic concern and medical competence, she forsook the couch in subsequent sessions and simply and poignantly confided her many anxieties as to her "advancing age," her fading beauty, her faithless husband, her ungrateful offspring, and the social ostracism to which she had increasingly been subjected because of her own defiantly flagrant extramarital adventures.

Therapy was correspondingly specific and direct: A period of disulfiram-reinforced abstinence from alcohol and a diminishing intake of drugs; a course at a beauty salon which restored much of her former attractiveness and led to greater sexual satisfactions in (and more discreetly outside) her marriage; a reutilization of her considerable artistic talents which led to a museum exhibition, and to a successful political campaign that helped restore her a position of social prestige and influence. Within 3 months the patient was relatively an emotionally stable, creative, and fairly happy woman who maintained this status during 2 years of follow-up.

### CASE 11: PSYCHOPHYSIOLOGIC (316.00)
### AND AFFECTIVE DISORDERS (300.40)
### WITH SCHIZOPHRENIC CHANNELIZATION (295.70)

Another patient epitomized regressive transitions from symbolically neurotic to depressive-regressive patterns, and then to dereism and suicide under ill-advised "therapy."

An eighteen-year-old girl was referred from the otolaryngology clinic because no organic reason could be found for her complaint of a constantly "dry and gravelly" throat which had made her avoid solid food during the preceding 2 months. The physical findings were completely normal except for a mild degree of undernourishment and secondary anemia.

The patient readily confided that she had many other physical complaints, such as blurred vision, "bad stomach," insomnia, and general muscular weakness. Of greater concern were an abhorrence of gasolinelike odors "which make my heart jump and I feel scared and like fainting," a fear of storms and of enclosed spaces, marked anxiety in heterosexual company, a conviction that she must never marry because "my children will be like me," and a growing melancholy with feelings of unworthiness, hopelessness, and suicidal preoccupations. The patient was hospitalized and the following additional history obtained:

She remembered her early childhood mainly in terms of frequent "storms" between her violently quarreling parents. The patient herself was antagonistic to her mother and highly partial to her father, with whom she was almost frankly erotic. As to her throat trouble, she remembered that when she was eight she suffered an attack of Vincent's angina for which her father, a house painter of limited means, had taken her to a famous and expensive clinic. She also clearly recalled the pleasure she felt after this in "scrubbing dad's back with gasoline to remove the paint caked on it," while he was taking his weekly bath.

At about the time of her menarche, an episode occurred indicating that early schizoid tendencies needed only relatively minor toxic and symbolic stimuli to find expression. One day the patient, after "accidentally" spilling some paint on herself, decided that she, too, needed to clean herself with gosoline, and actually bathed in the fluid. She became confused, ran into the street nude and there saw a vision of a patriarchial God, with features like her father, coming to crown her Queen of the Universe so she could summon "all women for judgment"; after this, she entered into a fuguelike state from which she could not be aroused for 2 days. No further hallucinatory episodes occurred, but she developed obsessions and compulsions, among them a fear of "closeness," countered by a desire "to touch everyone gently so that they would know that I really don't want to slap them." However, she managed to complete high school and to secure work in a bakery.

**Present Illness.** Six months before her admission, she had found a condom in her father's pocket, together with other evidence that he was conducting an extramarital liaison. Inasmuch as she had until then preferred to regard her father as somewhat of a saint, this discovery precipitated much brooding, during which she vaguely resolved that, if there was no virtue in the world, she too might as well dispense with her sexual inhibitions. Significantly, the person she selected for her first adventure was her employer, an elderly married man with few scruples about resisting her naively expressed invitations. However, her intended partner proved flaccid and, failing vaginal entry, suggested mutual exhibition and fellatio. At these requests the patient, who had been in a semitrance throughout the episode, entered into a state of dreamlike depersonalization from which she "awoke" only after her employer, himself in panic, had brought her home with the explanation that she "had begun acting crazy and then fainted." When a physician summoned by her father roused her with a strong whiff of ammonia, she complained that her vision was blurred and that she felt faint, and so weak that she could not open her mouth. These symptoms gradually improved under a regimen of bed rest, and "vitamin nerve tonics" administered morning and night by her father. But the "dry throat" and dysphagia persisted, and for these complaints she was referred to the Clinics.

**Course Under Therapy.** The patient demanded almost continuous attention on the ward, particularly from the senior psychiatrist, whom she would summon at odd hours "to tell him something else that's important." In general, her behavior was depressive: melancholic facies, prolonged, apparently unprovoked crying spells, slow movements, and the somatic accompaniments of anorexia, constipation and oligomenorrhea. Initial measures consisted of sedation, high caloric feeding, and the establishment of dyadic and group therapeutic relationships. In individual interviews, astonishingly frank "insights" appeared spontaneously: the patient equated her "fear of storms" with anxiety over "stormy" parental quarrels and fear of "closeness" with recollections of being confined in the bathroom with her nude father; so also, she associated her dysphagia directly with a "horrible impulse" she had experienced "to bite Mr.____'s (her employer's) penis off" when he had suggested fellatio. These fantasies were accepted, but were not encouraged or elaborated; instead, therapeutic emphasis was placed on the resumptions of realistic behavior. Within 3 weeks the patient showed improvement in mood and self-control; her appetite returned, she ate solid food (although significantly, she avoided meat), her vision cleared, she slept better, and regained a fair amount of energy and initiative. With help from her family, she was led to plan for a change of job, and enrolled in supervised social activities at her local synagogue. After 2 weeks of further improvement the patient, though still covertly obsessional on topics of sex, was free of physical complaints and was discharged—although with a guarded prognosis.

Our pessimism in this respect at first appeared unjustified, since the patient for several months seemed to adapt better in her familial relationships, worked steadily as a filing clerk in a small office, and cultivated a limited number of friends and social outlets under the gentle guidance of an elderly rabbi whom, predictably, she immediately venerated as a new embodiment of all virtue. However, a year after her discharge another and this time apparently quite minor sexual temptation precipitated a re-

turn of visual and gastric disturbances with compulsively ritualized behavior. Unfortunately, this time she was taken to a nonmedical self-styled "hypnotherapist" who treated her by daily
hours of "free association" under hypnosis. Within 2 weeks the
patient was again actively hallucinated and delusional; she was
convinced she had killed her father who, transformed into an
Avenging Angel, now "made her insides keep running out of
her vagina." The patient was committed to a state hospital and 6
months later, during a parole period at home, committed suicide.

## CASE 12: SCHIZOPHRENIA
## WITH SYMBOLIC DEREISM (295.14)

A twenty-eight-year-old woman was admitted with the complaints that she could not get rid of persistent ideas that she
"must not eat," was "going insane," or was "turning into a dog."
She had become unreasonably afraid of children and small animals, had developed various peculiar habits such as picking at
her hair until she was almost bald, holding onto a table while
kicking both legs backwards, and scrubbing out her mouth so often that the tissues were raw and bleeding.

**Anamnesis.** A combination of informants traced the patient's
disorder as follows:
She was one of four sisters, who (so they stated) had been
greatly attached to each other and to their mother—a person
who, according to them, existed only to serve her children. The
patient had done poorly in her studies, but had managed to get
through high school because of her conscientious attendance,
her reliability in performing tasks, and her subservience to the
nuns. However, these characteristics had made her unpopular
with her schoolmates, and she formed almost no social contacts
outside her family. The patient's mother died soon after the patient graduated from high school, and the father, who had long
considered himself unwanted by any of the women in his house,
promptly remarried and moved away.
The patient, after months of deep mourning for the

mother, transferred all her dependence to the eldest sister, and went to live in the latter's apartment. The sister, in overreaction to her previously strict compliance with maternal discipline, began to have affairs with various men, so that the patient once again felt displaced and homeless. In search of companionship and security, and naive in sexual matters, she, too, tried promiscuity for a time, became pregnant, and reluctantly married the father of her child. However, her husband was soon alienated by the patient's lack of personal warmth and her unending preoccupation with household trivialities. Moreover, although she spent much care and effort in feeding, dressing and training their daughter, the husband sensed that the strict routines and increasingly severe discipline imposed on the little girl indicated hostilities toward both him and his progeny. He therfore tried to compensate by special favoritism toward the child and avoided having more children by employing the only method of contraception permitted by his religion—sexual continence.

The patient became frigid and responded with increased sexual conflicts, whereupon the husband completed the cycle by seeking feminine warmth extramaritally. On one occasion when the patient was presented with evidence of his "unfaithfulness," she reacted with a visual experience in which her child, her husband, her home, and finally everything about her appeared small, as though displaced into the far distance. She was taken to an opthalmologist, who could find no organic signs of micropsia, but told the family that such symptoms sometimes occurred as the "first signs of a brain tumor." A neurologist also found no evidence of a somatic lesion, but the patient had already responded to the iatrogenic trauma with persistent fears that she was "going insane from brain disease," and therefore insisted that her child be taken care of by others to protect it from her possible "crazy impulses."

At this juncture, she found great surcrease in the rites and rituals of the Church, especially in long confessions in which she pleaded for and received forgiveness for "evil thoughts about my dear ones." She also sought to reestablish intimacy with her sisters, especially the eldest, with whom she tried to spend hours talking about the fondly remembered virtues of their mother. But eventually the priest warned her of "excessive scrupulosity," the sisters grew tired of her incessant demands, and from then on her deterioration was rapid. She developed a habit of kneeling repeatedly at home as though in silent prayer, yet instead of worshipful thoughts or words she mumbled inarticulate neologisms of doubt and reproach. Finally, her compulsive douching, mouthwashing, hair-picking (trichotilomania) and backward kicking necessitated her admission to the university hospital.

Here she presented a custodial problem, since she refused to rest or sleep adequately, and spent much of her time plying nurses, interns, other patients or even their visitors with the stock question: "Why do you think I can't have the right thoughts about Mr. _____ (her husband) and Ann (her daughter)"? Each time the patient did so she would apologize profusely but then repeat the question. She ate sparsely, and only with much urging, because of the insistent idea that food would cause her hair to grow "like an animal" and that eventually she "might turn into a dog." Similarly, any attempt to feed her by tube, keep her from pulling her hair out, or to confine her compulsive movements even in a continuous bath promptly induced such pathetic anxiety that these procedures had to be discontinued. To give her some measure of rest, therefore, she was kept under mild narcosis for several days (Chapter 13) and fed, conversed with, and given whatever reassurances seemed indicated while semiconscious.

It was during this period that the patient revealed some of the interrelationships of her phobias, obsessions, and compulsions. She recollected that when, during one of their quarrels, her husband had finally become exasperated and called her "a bitch," she admitted to herself that she was really "like a bitch" in that she had also performed fellatio—hence the mouthwashing; also the necessity to tear the hair off her head and body so that she "would look as little like an animal as possible." Since all sex was also "dirty" and "like an animal," she had felt impelled to kick her legs out backward "like a bitch chasing away dogs"—a reaction which made her husband regret his angry epithet. While recounting such fantasies the patient would often berate herself "for making so much trouble for my good, good husband and my sweet little girl"—but at the same time she would reveal her covert gratification by her gestures and facial expressions; similarly, while deploring her inexorable fate ("I'll be put away forever in a mental hospital.") she also implied a regressive desire to escape into a fantasied haven of irresponsibility and dependence.

**Course.**Under benzodiazepines and phenothiazine medication her symptoms were partially controlled, at which point her sisters demanded her discharge. Once home, however, she refused further medication, whereupon her bizarre behavior recurred. She also became hallucinated and delusional, saw and heard animal-like figures that threatened her sexually, and felt herself actually "turning into a dog from the waist down." At a state hospital she was given 18 electroshock convulsive treatments which again controlled her acutely psychotic behavior; but the patient became so slovenly, amnestic, and lacking in initiative that permanent custodial care has since become necessary.

### CASE 13: HYPOMANIA FOLLOWING A PROLONGED DEPRESSION (301.13)

The following patient, although not typical of a genetically or neurochemically determined manic-depressive psychoses, nevertheless illustrates the psychodynamic and therapeutic vectors operative in many if not all such syndromes.

A wealthy executive aged fifty-two was brought to the hospital by a business associate who stated that the patient "had been running himself so ragged with too much work and too much play" that his friends had insisted that he come to the university for "a checkup and a rest-cure." Questioning revealed that for the preceding 4 months the patient had been working intensely but erratically, making quick business decisions that sometimes produced brilliant results, but as often proved unsound. His social behavior had also become impulsive and unpredictable; for instance, he had twice abruptly adjourned business conferences in the midst of serious deliberations with an abrupt invitation to everyone present to "quit, have a drink, and come play golf at my club." On the first occasion a few present had good-naturedly accepted, but while he was driving them to the golf course he suddenly expanded his invitation to include a weekend for everyone at his country home 200 miles away, and had with difficulty been dissuaded from heading there immediately. The patient's impetuosity, restlessness, extravagance, excessive drinking, and forced gaiety had increasingly concerned his friends, who had previously considered him a sober, stable, and rather undemonstrative individual.

In the hospital the patient's behavior appeared pseudomanic. He dressed in flashy pajamas and loud bathrobes and was otherwise immodest and careless about his personal appearance. He neglected his meals and rest hours, and was irregular and distractible in his adaptations to routine. Without apparent intent to be disturbing he sang, whistled, told pointless off-color stories and visited indiscriminately and flirted crudely with the nurses and female patients. Superficially, he appeared to be in high spirits, and yet one day when he was being gently chided over some particularly irresponsible act he suddenly slumped in a chair, covered his face with his hands, began sobbing, and cried, "For God's sake, doc, let me be. Can't you see that I've just *got* to act happy?"

This reversal of mood was transient and his surface buoyancy returned in a few moments; nevertheless, during a sodium amytal interview, his seeming euphoria again dropped away and he burst into frank sobbing as he clung to the physician's arm. He then confided that during the preceding year he had begun to suspect, with some reason, that his young second wife whom he "loved to distraction" had tired of their marriage and had been unfaithful to him. He had accused her of this, and she had replied with a callous offer of divorce. His pride had been greatly wounded, but to salvage it, avoid the scandal of a second divorce, and keep her as long as possible, they had agreed that she take an extended European tour and postpone her decision until her return. During her absence he had been obsessively torn by suspense, jealousy, and anger, could no longer take an interest in his work, and had lost sleep, strength, and weight. He consulted his family physician for the latter symptoms but the doctor, after finding little physically wrong with him, had simply advised him "to forget your business (sic) troubles, play a bit more golf, get about more and enjoy yourself." He had followed this advice with compulsive intensity, but with the abreactive exaggeration that had evenually led to his admission to the hospital.

This account served to initiate further confidences. In subsequent interviews, the patient also "confessed" that during the past several years he had begun to feel that his place near the head of a business concern was being threatened by younger, more energetic, and better-trained men, in competition with whom he himself had thought it necessary to become ultra-"progressive" in his executive tasks. In private life, too, he had become afraid of being considered "just a nice old has-been," and had therefore begun to indulge in drinking, stag-party venery, and marital irresponsibilities that had caused his first divorce 3 years previously. In his continued denial of feared obsolescence, he had contracted a second marriage a year later to a young, pretty, and popular widow whom he had, by offering her a life of wealth and ease, won away from more youthful admirers. However, in his anxiety also to prove his sexual competence, he had frequently been impotent with her, and had then made their marriage almost intolerable by his reactive rages and jealousies. As a result, she had very probably become unfaithful and was currently spending more of his money in Europe in anticipation of an eventual separation.

**Therapy.** Under a 3-week regimen of proper diet, relaxing physiotherapy, mild sedation (lithium and tricyclics were not administered), and calming group sessions the pseudomanic behavior abated. Reorientative psychotherapy then dealt with the following issues: (a) that despite his recent excesses, he had retained the physical and mental capacities and business skills that still made him a valuable asset to his company (a point on which the therapist had been assured)[3]; (b) that since his social and financial positions were as yet relatively unimpaired, it would very likely be in his wife's interest to renew their trial at marriage; (c) that joint counselling would then help resolve their mutual distrusts, leading to enhanced sexual compatibility; and (d) with personal, marital, and career securities thus reasonably restored, he could resume a relatively sober and stable style of life. When his wife returned from abroad, these issues were further clarified to her interim satisfaction. The couple was then followed in weekly and then biweekly outpatient interviews for 3 months, after which occasional contacts during the ensuing 2 years indicated that they had attained about an average degree of upper middle-class contentment, with no return of the patient's serious aberrations of behavior.

### CASE 14: PSYCHOGENIC PAIN DISORDER (307.80)

A fifty-four-year-old spinster complained that the right side of her face and neck was affected by severe pains, the cause of which could not be determined by physical and laboratory examinations, and which persisted despite all medication. The psychiatric history revealed that the patient had but one friend—a neighbor whose husband 6 months previously had developed a malignant right cervical tumor. On the patient's urging, he had been taken to the university hospital, where he died in a few weeks. The patient's friend, in her depth of grief, had turned furiously on the patient with the accusations that the latter had "sent him to die" and that, had she not done so, he would still be alive. Soon after this scene the patient herself developed facial pains very like those of the deceased husband, and promptly entered the university hospital with the emphatic statement that she herself was certain it was "the best hospital in the country." Other data revealed a less conscious dynamism than this relatively simple one of self-justification: the attachment of the two women friends had long been homosexual, and the patient was symbolically identifying with the dead husband.

Therapy consisted of reassurances to the patient that "nervous pains" in any part of the body could be caused by "worry and aggravation," and concurrent reexplanations to the widow that her husband's illness had been inevitably fatal despite the best of treatment. Once a reconciliation between the women had been effected, the patient's pains responded promptly to placebos and mild massage and she was discharged symptom-free.

### CASE 15: GERIATRIC PERSONALITY DISORDER (292.89); THERAPEUTIC REHABILITATION

A seventy-year-old patient, before his retirement, had been very successful as the owner of a string of cigar factories. After a half decade of idleness or aimless travel, he had begun to drink, gamble, and—perhaps with not altogether unconscious intent —"disgrace" his protesting children with various escapades until, by legal threats, they forced him to seek treatment. The therapist abjured the role of parole officer, actively cultivated the patient's confidence, and professed genuine interest in the social implications of his "pioneer contributions to American industry"—particularly as to how he had eliminated marginal labor by substituting machines for cigar-rolling Puerto Ricans. This encouraged the patient to regale the therapist with instructive lectures on commerce and finance. During one such session, he vowed to retaliate for alleged poor service and discourtesies at a local cigar counter by starting a string of tobacco-and-notion dispensaries in downtown buildings which, predictably, were to feature the products of the various factories that still bore his name. He was encouraged to do so, and once started on this project he was, almost to his death 8 years later, a sometimes assertive and irascible, but mostly alert, active, useful, certainly more likable and undoubtedly happier senior citizen.

### CASE 16: FAMILY THERAPY; FORENSIC ASPECTS (V71.01)

A forty-two-year-old systems accountant was referred by an industrial firm with the comment "Mr. W.Z. who has been a valuable employee for the past 21 years, is under indictment for sexual abuse to his step-daughter. Please advise." Mr. Z., a spare, stooped, prematurely wizened person, was manifestly suffering from an intense depression and readily confessed to suicidal preoccupations. He tendered the following history:

Raised with four older siblings in a repressively religious and essentially loveless family, he had felt isolated and alienated during his schooling, had developed few esthetic or recreational interests and had concentrated on his only talent: a ready grasp of mathematics and accounting. After two years of technical training he had secured his present employment as a computer technician and had served his employers reasonably well for two decades but, again because of his self-effacing and constricted relationships with peers and supervisors, he had not been advanced to managerial or other responsibilities.

Twenty years ago, after a series of sexual frustrations, he had married "the only girl I thought would ever consider living with me"; however, the childless marriage had ended in divorce five years later because of his affective inhibitions, her sexual frigidity and her dissatisfaction with his lack of social grace or economic advancement. Mr. Z. then spent another lonesome eight years before marrying a troubled 45-year-old divorcee with an 11-year-old daughter. The girl, who had been starved for affection from both her natural parents even before their divorce three years previously, found her new stepfather avidly receptive of her overtures for attention. Mr. Z. was again treated with growing indifference by the second Mrs. Z., and in compensation he "let the child, whenever she wanted to, sit on my lap and hug me a little to show she loved her new daddy." Predictably, as she grew older some of the attendant contrectation, although it never approached genital contacts, began to assume mutually erotic undertones, leading to the following serious consequences:

During the week preceeding Mr. Z's referral, the girl's class had been subjected to a series of pejorative lectures by the school psychologist on the devastating effects of parental "sex abuses" and the absolute necessity of "reporting them immediately to the authorities". The daughter described her experiences to the psychologist, who conveyed them then to the school principal, who as promptly relayed them, apparently with sensational elaborations, to the district attorney. The latter, with a special zeal springing from some recently publicized failures in his other functions, promptly arrested Mr. Z. and personally threatened him with a jury trial and seven years of imprisonment. Mr. Z. engaged a defense attorney, but received scant comfort from the latter's assurance that he "would try for the minimum sentence of just one year, because both the district prosecutor and judge are out to get sex fiends." After four anorexic days, sleepless nights and obvious exhaustion Mr. Z. was sent by his supervisor to the company's medical department and, in obviously desperate straits, readily accepted psychiatric consultation.

## Therapy.

This consisted of separate interviews with the wife and child, followed by a family session:

*The Wife.* The second Mrs. Z. confided that she had been increasingly resentful of her husband's characteristic "aloofness" and "lack of progress"—and, as could be surmised, also jealous of her daughter's budding sexual behavior. She seemed initially indifferent to her husband's fate: however when, in all objectivity, we discussed how his incarceration would also entail highly adverse economic, social and other consequences for her and her daughter, she promised "to talk to the girl to see what we should do."

*The Child.* Miss Z., a tearful, confused and seriously troubled adolescent, was at first convinced she could not extricate herself from a hopeless situation because the district attorney had, with her naive consent, videotaped her accounts of how "daddy had hugged and kissed and patted me while we watched TV together every night." However, she responded eagerly to a gentle, avuncular approach, and listened intelligently and receptively to these options as outlined for her:

If, because of her accusations, her father went to jail, she would not only be deprived of economic support, but also feel guilty about sending him there, be subject to often cruel derisions from her schoolmates for being "the daughter of a criminal", be more vulnerable to sexual advances from "boyfriends", and suffer other regrets and difficulties about which it was my obligation to inform her as a physician concerned with her welfare.

However, while I could not advise her to change her testimony (since it might be considered subornation) she could also inform the prosecuting attorney that if forced to testify in court, she could honestly say that she had always welcomed her stepfather's affection, had never considered herself "sexually abused" and had truthfully felt she was being happily and morally raised by both her present parents.

*The Family Interview.* With the consent of both mother and daughter the above issues were reviewed and clarified. The mother—and not I—then began to urge the daughter to "straighten out this mess for everybody's sake" and the daughter, still tearful, but crestfallen and contrite, agreed to do so. With obvious relief on the part of the father, the family requested further counseling after the trial ten days hence.

*Follow-up.* Two weeks later I was informed by Mr. Z.'s company physician that the district attorney had dropped all charges and that Mr. Z. had returned to productive employment. The girl had changed schools, and the family now "wished the whole affair forgotten" and therefore had declined further counseling—the latter a not altogether favorable development.

## NOTES

1. A detailed account of the successful psychoanalysis of a patient with severe anorexia nervosa will be found in Masserman, 1946, Appendix I. For a plethora of other case histories, legal opinions, insurance reports, and other clinical illustrations, see Masserman, 1955.

2. This understandable lack of concern about a symptomatic disability that serves to resolve a neurotic conflict was called "*la belle indifference*" by Janet; but the underlying anxiety can be readily elicited if the symptom is prematurely threatened by the therapist.

3. If the patient also had a history of previous "breakdowns" (other than his overreactions to his divorce) or if there had been current evidences of alcoholic or other physical deterioration, the therapy would have been more complicated and the prognosis less favorable.

*Chapter 16*

# REVIEW AND INTEGRATION

Human beings have historically sought the following universal and ultimate (Ur) objectives (Chapters 1 and 2):

  I.  *Physical*: for strength, survival and procreation,
 II.  *Social*: for interpersonal securities, and
III.  *Metaphsychologic*: for beliefs in supernatural systems wishfully conceived and controlled.

But since our attainments have ever been illusory and asymptotic, our resultant anxieties and concomitant aberrations of behavior have required meliorative individual, group, and existential services. Physicians and other health therapists have served (Greek *therapeien,* service) in these respects as follows:

**Communications.** Empathetic exchanges of views (interviews) and examinations have led to comprehensive appraisals (diagnoses) of the patient's past somatic, social, and philosophic maladaptations (Chapters 3 and 4) that eventuated in his respective current difficulties.

**Therapies.** The patient's travails have then been mitigated by various somatic, dyadic, behavioral, and group modalities (Chapters 5–15), the dynamics of which could be reduced to the following therapeutic parameters:

1. The initial *reputation* of the therapist as a competent specialist, potential friend and philosophic mentor,
2. The cultivation of *rapport* enhanced by
3. The *relief* of the patient's physical, social, or existential discomforts through optimal combinations of environmental, medical, dyadic, and group therapies,
4. A *review* of (a) the nature and severity of the stresses that exacerbated the patient's maladaptations, (b) the preceding constitutional and experiential factors that rendered him vulnerable and (c) his resources of talents, intelligence, skills, and coping capacities, eventuating in
5. Mutually acceptable *reorientations* of the patient's motivations, perceptions, values, and goals, as applied to
6. *Rehabilitative* applications toward a more adaptive, creative, and ultimately happier life, followed by
7. A *recycling* of the above whenever desired.

Throughout, therapy is expedited by:

Assurances of complete confidentiality except when communications with others become essential for the patient's interests.

A practicable schedule of sessions with the patient and others as needed.

Individuation of techniques in accord with the patients' somatic state, educational and occupational levels, intelligence, and ethnic or cultural orientations and other relevant vectors.

Concentration on the patient's behavior in the here and now, with anamnestic tracings sufficient only to clarify retained but inapt childhood and adolescent patterns.

Acceptance of the reality that whatever the patient's rationalizations (as to his "genetic proclivities . . . unconscious
complexes . . childhood conditioning . . . ingrained habits," etc.) he will be held accountable for his conduct by
society and in one way or another be penalized or rewarded accordingly.

**Results.** The author has elsewhere reviewed in detail the vast
literature on the methods, controls, statistical manipulations,
and evaluative cautions required to assay the desired versus the
adverse effects of different modalities of therapy as applied to a
great variety of patients. His inferences were that whenever any
form of treatment, irrespective of its professed rationale and
technique, was conducted in approximate accord with the therapeutic parameters outlined above and thereby fulfilled one or
more of the patient's UR-needs, the results compared favorably
with those obtained in any other medical or allied speciality
(Masserman, 1982, pp. 20-33.).

## MULTUM IN PARVO

Man's Ur-anxieties are triune: his abhorence of illness and
death; his doubts as to his social securities; and his fears of being
a cosmic triviality. These triple trepidations motivate three compensatory maneuvers: his attempts to subjugate his milieu
through his sciences and technologies, his efforts to guarantee
his familial, economic, and political alliances, and his endeavors
to encompass the universe in his philosophic and religious systems. Unfortunately, his strivings in all these modalities often
fail, whereupon he becomes an impatient patient and calls upon
dedicated professionals to redress his frustrations. The services
required are again tripartite: the restoration of bodily strengths
and skills, the recultivation of secure human relationships, and
the restoration of transcendant faiths. How each therapist, acting as physician, social ombudsman and philosophic mentor
combines these therapeutic influences constitutes his or her clinical artistry.
Can mortal beings do more?

*APPENDIX I*

# DIAGNOSTIC AND STATISTICAL MANUAL OF THE AMERICAN PSYCHIATRIC ASSOCIATION, 3RD ED.[1]

All official DSM-III codes and terms are included in ICD-9.[2] However, in order to differentiate those DSM-III categories that use the same ICD-9-CM codes, unofficial non-ICD-9-CM codes are provided in parentheses for use when greater specificity is necessary.

### DISORDERS USUALLY FIRST EVIDENT IN INFANCY, CHILDHOOD, OR ADOLESCENCE

#### Mental Retardation

(Code in fifth digit: 1 = with other behavioral symptoms (requiring attention or treatment and that are not part of another disorder), 0 = without other behavioral symptoms.)

317.0 (x) Mild mental retardation

318.0 (x) Moderate mental retardation

318.1 (x) Severe mental retardation

318.2 (x) Profound mental retardation

319.0 (x) Unspecified mental retardation

### Attention Deficit Disorder

314.01 with hyperactivity
314.00 without hyperactivity
314.80 residual type

### Conduct Disorder

312.00 undersocialized, aggressive
312.10 undersocialized, nonaggressive
312.23 socialized, aggressive
312.21 socialized, nonaggressive
312.90 atypical

### Anxiety Disorders of Childhood or Adolescence

309.21 Separation anxiety disorder
313.21 Avoidant disorder of childhood or adolescence
313.00 Overanxious disorder

### Other Disorders of Infancy, Childhood or Adolescence

313.89 Reactive attachment disorder of infancy
313.22 Schizoid disorder of childhood or adolescence
313.23 Elective mutism
313.81 Oppositional disorder
313.82 Identity disorder

### Eating Disorders

307.10 Anorexia nervosa    307.53 Rumination disorder of in -
   fancy
307.51 Bulimia    307.50 Atypical eating disorder
307.52 Pica

### Stereotyped Movement Disorders

307.21 Transient tic disorder
307.22 Chronic motor tic disorder

307.23 Tourette's disorder

307.20 Atypical tic disorder

307.30 Atypical stereotyped movement disorder

### Other Disorders with Physical Manifestations

307.00 Stuttering    307.60 Functional enuresis

307.70 Functional encopresis

307.46 Sleepwalking disorder

307.46 (307.49) Sleep terror disorder

### Pervasive Development Disorders

Code in fifth digit: 0 = full syndrome present, 1-residual state.

299.0x Infantile autism

299.8x Childhood onset pervasive developmental disorder

299.9x Atypical

### Specific Developmental Disorders. Note: These are coded on Axis II.

315.00 Developmental reading disorder

315.10 Developmental arithmetic disorder

315.31 Developmental language disorder

315.39 Developmental articulation disorder

315.50 Mixed specific developmental disorder

315.90 Atypical specific developmental disorder

### ORGANIC MENTAL DISORDERS

Section 1. Organic mental disorders whose etiology or pathophysiological process is listed below (taken from the mental disorders section of ICD-9-CM).

### Senile and Presenile Dementias

Primary degenerative dementia, senile onset.

290.30 with delirium

290.20 with delusions

290.21 with depression

290.00 uncomplicated

Code in fifth digit: 0 = uncomplicated, 1 = with delirium, 2 = with delusions, 3 = with depression.

290.1x Primary degenerative dementia, presenile onset

290.4x Multi-infarct dementia

### Substance-induced

*Alcohol*

303.00 intoxication

291.40 idiosyncratic intoxication

291.80 withdrawal

291.00 withdrawal delirium

291.30 hallucinosis   291.10 amnestic disorder

Code severity of dementia in fifth digit: 1 = mild, 2 = moderate, 3 = severe, 0 = unspecified.

291.2x Dementia associated with alcoholism, barbiturate or similarly acting sedative or hypnotic

305.40 intoxication (327.00)

292.00 withdrawal (327.01)

292.00 withdrawal delirium (327.02)

292.83 amnestic disorder (327.04)

*Opioid*

305.50 intoxication (327.10)   292.00 withdrawal (327.11)

*Cocaine*

305.60 intoxication (327.20)

*Amphetamine or Similarly Acting Sympathomimetic*

305.70 intoxication (327.30)

292.81 delirium (327.32)   292.11 delusional disorder (327.35)

292.00 withdrawal (327.31)

*Phencyclidine (PCP) or Similarly Acting Arylcyclo-hexylamine*

305.90 intoxication (327.40) 292.81 delirium (327.42)

292.80 mixed organic mental disorder (327.49)

*Hallucinogen*

305.30 hallucinosis (327.5)

292.11 delusional disorder (327.55)

292.84 affective disorder (327.57)

*Cannabis*

305.20 intoxication (327.60)

292.11 delusional disorder (327.65)

*Tobacco*

292.00 withdrawal (327.71)

*Caffeine*

305.90 intoxication (327.80)

*Other or Unspecified Substance*

305.90 intoxication (327.90)

292.00 withdrawal (327.91)    292.81 delirium (327.92)

292.82 dementia (327.93)    292.83 amnestic disorder (327.94)

292.11 delusional disorder (327.95) 292.12 hallucinosis (327.96)

292.84 affective disorder (327.97)

292.89 personality disorder (327.98)

292.90 atypical or mixed organic mental disorder (327.99)

Section 2. Organic brain syndromes whose etiology or pathophysiological process is either noted as an additional diagnosis from outside the mental disorders section of ICD-9-CM or is unknown.

293.00 Delirium   294.10 dementia

294.00 Amnestic syndrome   293.81 Organic delusional syndrome

293.82 Organic hallucinosis   293.83 Organic affective syndrome

310.10 Organic personality syndrome

294.80 Atypical or mixed organic brain syndrome

## SUBSTANCE USE DISORDERS

Code in fifth digit: 1 = continuous, 2-episodic, 3 = in remission, 0 = unspecified.

305.0x Alcohol abuse

303.9x Alcohol dependence (Alcoholism)

305.4x Barbiturate or similarly acting sedative or hypnotic abuse

304.1x Barbiturate or similarly acting sedative or hypnotic dependence

305.5x Opioid abuse

304.0X Opioid dependence

305.6x Cocaine abuse

305.7x Amphetamine or similarly acting sympathomimetic abuse

304.4x Amphetamine or similarly acting sympathomimetic dependence

305.9x Phencyclidine (PCP) or similarly acting arylcyclohexylamine abuse (328.4x)

305.3x Hallucinogen abuse

305.2x Cannabis abuse

304.3x Cannabis dependence

305.1x Tobacco dependence

305.9x Other, mixed or unspecified substance abuse

304.6x Other specified substance dependence
304.9x Unspecified substance dependence
304.7x Dependence on combination of opioid and other nonalcoholic substance
304.8x Dependence on combination of substances, excluding opioids and alcohol

### SCHIZOPHRENIC DISORDERS

Code in fifth digit: 1 = subchronic, 2 = chronic, 3 = subchronic with acute exacerbation, 4 = chronic with acute exacerbation, 5 = in remission, 0 = unspecified.

#### Schizophrenia

295.1x disorganized    295.2x catatonic
295.3x paranoid    295.9x undifferentiated
295.6x residual

### PARANOID DISORDERS

297.10 Paranoia    297.30 Shared paranoid disorder
298.30 Acute paranoid disorder 297.90 Atypical paranoid disorder

### PSYCHOTIC DISORDERS NOT ELSEWHERE CLASSIFIED

295.40 Schizophreniform disorder
298.80 Brief reactive psychosis
296.70 Schizoaffective disorder    298.90 Atypical psychosis

### NEUROTIC DISORDERS

These are included in Affective, Anxiety, Somatoform, Dissociative, and Psychosexual Disorders. In order to facilitate the identification of the categories that in DSM-II were grouped together in the class of Neuroses, the DSM-II terms are included separately in parentheses after the corresponding categories. These DSM-II terms are included in ICD-9-CM and therefore are acceptable as alternatives to the recommended DSM-III terms that precede them.

## AFFECTIVE DISORDERS

### Major Affective Disorders

Code major depressive episode in fifth digit: 6 = in remission, 4 = with psychotic features (the unofficial non-ICD-9-CM fifth digit 7 may be used instead to indicate that the psychotic features are mood-incongruent), 3 = with melancholia, 2 = without melancholia, 0 = unspecified.

Code manic episode in fifth digit: 6 = in remission, 4 = with psychotic features (the unofficial non-ICD-9-CM fifth digit 7 may be used instead to indicate that the psychotic features are mood-incongruent), 2 = without psychotic features, 0 = unspecified.

#### *Bipolar Disorder*

296.6x mixed
296.4x manic
296.5x depressed
Major depression    296.2x single episode
                    296.3x recurrent

#### *Other Specific Affective Disorders*

301.13 Cyclothymic disorder
300.40 Dysthymic disorder (or Depressive neurosis)

#### *Atypical Affective Disorders*

296.70 Atypical bipolar disorder    296.82 Atypical depression

### ANXIETY DISORDERS

## Phobic Disorders (or Phobic Neuroses)

300.21 Agoraphobia with panic attacks
300.22 Agoraphobia without panic attacks
300.23 Social phobia   300.29 Simple phobia

## Anxiety States (or Anxiety Neuroses)

300.01 Panic disorder   300.02 Generalized anxiety disorder
300.30 Obsessive compulsive disorder (or Obsessive neurosis)

*Post-Traumatic Disorder*

308.30 acute   309.81 chronic or delayed
300.00 Atypical anxiety disorder

### SOMATOFORM DISORDERS

300.81 Somatization disorder
300.11 Conversion disorder (or Hysterical neurosis, conversion
type)   307.80 Psychogenic pain disorder
300.70 Hypochondriasis (or Hypochondriacal neurosis)
300.71 Atypical somatoform disorder

### DISSOCIATIVE DISORDERS (OR HYSTERICAL NEUROSES, DISSOCIATIVE TYPE)

300.12 Psychogenic amnesia   300.13 Psychogenic amnesia
300.14 Multiple personality   300.60 Depersonalization disorder (or Depersonalization neurosis)
300.15 Atypical dissociative disorder

## PSYCHOSEXUAL DISORDERS

### Gender Identity Disorders

Indicate sexual history in the fifth digit of Transsexualism code:
1 = asexual, 2 = homosexual, 3 = heterosexual, 0 = unspecified.

302.5x Transsexualism
302.60 Gender identity disorder of childhood
302.85 Atypical gender identity disorder

### Paraphilias

302.81 Fetishism    302.30 Transvestism
302.10 Zoophilia    302.20 Pedophilia
302.40 Exhibitionism    302.82 Voyeurism
302.83 Sexual masochism    302.84 Sexual sadism
302.89 Atypical paraphilia

### Psychosexual Dysfunctions

302.71 Inhibited sexual desire    302.72 Inhibited sexual excitement
302.73 Inhibited female orgasm    302.74 Inhibited male orgasm
302.75 Premature ejaculation    302.76 Functional dyspareunia
306.51 Functional vaginismus    302.79 Atypical psychosexual dysfunction

### Other Psychosexual Disorders

302.00 Ego-dystonic homosexuality
302.90 Psychosexual disorder not elsewhere classified

## FACTITIOUS DISORDERS

300.16 Factitious disorder with psychological symptoms
301.51 Chronic factitious disorder with physical symptoms
300.19 Atypical factitious disorder with physical symptoms

## DISORDERS OF IMPULSE CONTROL NOT ELSEWHERE CLASSIFIED

312.31 Pathological gambling    312.32 Kleptomania
312.33 Pyromania    312.33 Intermittent explosive disorder
312.35 Isolated explosive disorder    312.39 Atypical impulse control disorder

## ADJUSTMENT DISORDER

309.00 with depressed mood    309.24 with anxious mood
309.28 with mixed emotional features
309.30 with disturbance of conduct
309.40 with mixed disturbance of emotions and conduct
309.23 with work (or academic) inhibition
309.83 with withdrawal
309.90 with atypical features

## PSYCHOLOGICAL FACTORS AFFECTING PHYSICAL CONDITION

Specify physical condition on Axis III.
316.00 Psychological factors affecting physical condition.

## PERSONALITY DISORDERS

Note: These are coded on Axis II

301.00 Paranoid    301.20 Schizoid    301.22 Schizotypal
301.50 Histronic    301.81 Narcissistic
301.70 Antisocial    301.83 Borderline
301.82 Avoidant    301.60 Dependent
301.40 Compulsive    301.84 Passive-Aggressive
301.89 Atypical, mixed, or other personality disorder

### CODES FOR CONDITIONS NOT ATTRIBUTABLE TO A
### MENTAL DISORDER THAT ARE A FOCUS OF
### ATTENTION OR TREATMENT

V65.20 Malingering    V62.89 Borderline intellectual functioning (V62.88)

V71.01 Adult antisocial behavior

V71.02 Childhood or adolescent antisocial behavior

V62.30 Academic problem

V62.20 Occupational problem

V62.82 Uncomplicated bereavement

V15.80 Noncompliance with medical treatment

V62.89 Phase of life problem or other life circumstance problem

V61.10 Marital problem    V61.20 Parent-child problem

V61.80 Other specified family circumstances

V62.81 Other interpersonal problem

### ADDITIONAL CODES

300.99 Unspecified mental disorder (nonpsychotic)

V71.07 No diagnosis or condition on Axis I

799.91 Diagnosis or condition deferred on Axis I

V71.08 No diagnosis on Axis II

799.92 Diagnosis deferred on Axis II

### SUPPLEMENTARY AXES

I DSM III classification; II Personality factors; III Organic disease; IV Recent stresses; V Decompensation in past year. Degree of dysfunction graded 0 to 5.

### NOTES

1. Reproduced by kind permission of Dr. Melvin Sabshin, Medical Director, American Psychiatric Association. For a critique, see chapter 4.

2. International Classification of Diseases, 9th ed., with annotations.

# GLOSSARY
## An Alphabetical Review of Theory, Symptomatology, Diagnosis, and Therapy

*Affect:*Generalized feeling tone, usually distinguished from emotion in being more persistent and pervasive, less intensely reflected physiologically and with more generalized ideational content.

*Akathisia:* Urgency to restless muscular activity, such as may be induced by neuroleptic drugs.

*Alzheimer's Disease:*Severe presenile or senile mental and behavioral deterioration due to cerebral fibrillosis.

*Ambivalence:* Incompatibility of covert motivations with regard to alternate possibilities of action; e.g., mixed love and hate for the same person.

*Amentia:* Lack of development of intellectual (q.v.) capacities, due to congenital defects.

*Amnesia:* Loss of memory or recall. *Retrograde* a. signifies forgetfulness for events preceding some *amnemonic trauma* such as cerebral concussion or an epileptic seizure, as distinguished from *anterograde a.*, or loss of memory for following events. *Lacunar* or *patchy a.* connotes an inability to recall specific events or portions of them, with preserved memory for episodes between them.

*Anaclisis*:Dependent leaning on a person.

*Anhedonia*:Inability to experience pleasure.

*Anima*:The unconscious feminine nidus in men (C. Jung).

*Animus:* The unconscious male nidus in women (C. Jung).

*Anorexia Nervosa*: Prolonged neurotic self-starvation; usually in young women, with amenorrhea, sexual frigidity, and progressive cachexia.

*Anxiety*:A state of apprehensive tension which arises during adaptational conflicts and insecurities. Anxiety is experienced in circumstances connoting symbolic danger, or when phobic, compulsive, paranoid, or other accustomed adaptations are transgressed. A. may stimulate solutions of problems, or rise to *panic*.

*Anxiety Syndrome*:The physiologic concomitants of anxiety, generally experienced as palpitation (consciousness of racing or pounding heart), shallow, rapid, or constricted respiration, globus (sensations of tightness or lump in the throat), trembling, "fluttering" in the abdomen, sweaty, flushed or pale skin, and a diffuse apprehensiveness which may mount to feelings of impending catastrophe. Incontinence may occur in severe episodes.

*Aphasia*: Impairment of communicative functions. *Sensory* or *impressive a.* denotes impaired recall (*amnestic a.*) recognition (*anomia*), or correlation (*syntactic a.*) of speech symbols; *motor expressive a.* indicates a loss of verbal, written, or mimetic speech. These types of a. are all present in varying degree in *organic a.* and, when complete, constitute *global a.* In *functional* or *neurotic* (q.v.) *a*. one or several of the above dysfunctions may appear in relative isolation.

*Apraxia*:Loss of motor skills.

*Association, Free*:1. The psychoanalytic technique of requiring the patient to express or describe all thoughts, sensations, and emotions as they occur during the analytic hour. 2. The verbalizations so elicited.

*Aura*: Sensations or other prodromal experiences (sometimes hallucinatory) which regularly or irregularly precede each episode of a paroxysmal disorder; e.g., migraine or epilepsy (q.v.).

*Automatism*:Mechanical, repetitious, apparently undirected, symbolic behavior, often without conscious control; seen in fugue states or schizophrenia (q.v.).

*Autonomic Nervous System*:The portion of the nervous system that regulates the glands, circulation, and internal organs. Its *parasympathetic* (cranosacral) division is in general anabolic and inhibitory; its *orthosympathetic* (thoraco-lumbar) division is in general catabolic and excitatory, but there are specific exceptions in organ-innervation, and the two divisions are intimately interactive.

*Behaviorism*:A system of psychology that studies the conduct of human beings exclusively on the principle of association and professes to exclude consciousness and other subjective and conative considerations as irrelevant epiphenomena (Chapter 10).

*Bestiality*: Sexual intercourse with animals.

*Biodynamics*:The historical, comparative, and experimental study of the genetic, environmental, experiential, and therapeutic dynamics which determine the behavior of organisms (Chapters 1 and 5).

*Briquet Syndrome:*Formerly hysteria, q.v.

*Bulimia:*Excessive hunger and food intake.

*Castration Complex:*In psychoanalytic theory, fear of traumatic degenitalization in either sex as punishment for forbidden erotic desires. The term, however, has been used with a variety of connotations ranging from fear of literal castration (Freud) to symbolic deprivation of any cherished possession (Chapter 8).

*Cataplexy:*A transient attack of muscular weakness with or without loss of consciousness. May occur in conjunction with narcolepsy (q.v.).

*Catastrophic Reaction:*Severe disintegration of behavior under excessive stress, especially in patients whose adaptive capacities are impaired by cerebral injury (K. Goldstein).

*Catatonia:*A clinical form of *schizophrenia* (q.v.) characterized by *negativism* (q.v.), motor rigidity, or, rarely *flexibilitas cerea*, stupor, occasional marked excitement, and an episodic course (Chapter 4).

*Catharsis:*The partial dissipation of the morbid residuals of a repressed traumatic experience by therapeutic verbalization or *acting-out,* accompanied by an emotional discharge or *abreaction.* This occurs during psychoanalytic therapy, or it may be induced by hypnosis (*hypnocatharsis*) or drugs (*narcoanalysis*) with or without interpretation and guided retraining by the therapist (*narcosynthesis*)—a form of rapid therapy often effective in acute combat neuroses (V. Horsley, R. Grinker).

*Cathexis:*In psychoanalysis, "libidinal charge," or investment of an object or idea with special significance or value-tone; e.g., individualized love, hatred, or ambivalent combinations of affect with reference to a thing or person.

*Character:*The interrelated patterns of behavior of an individual; distinguished by some from *personality,* in that the latter may mean more specifically the social manifestations of character patterns.

*Community Mental Health*: Preventive and therapeutic psychiatric programs in collaboration with allied disciplines and social agencies (Chapter 11).

*Complex, Inferiority*: In Adlerian individual psychology, covert feelings of incompetence stemming from excessive disciplinary subordination or physical inadequacies (*organ inferiority*) in childhood, for which the individual may try to overcompensate by excessive ambitiousness, aggressiveness, domination, or special accomplishment.

*Complex, Oedipus*: In early psychoanalytic theory, the erotic attachment of the child to the parent of the opposite sex, repressed because of the fear of *castration* (q.v.) by the jealous parent (Chapters 2 and 8). (From the Greek in which Laius, King of Thebes, exiles his infant son Oedipus, who is rescued by a shepherd. Later, Oedipus in his wanderings [identity seeking] unknowingly kills his father and marries Jocasta, his mother. When he discovers this, he blinds [symbolically castrates] himself, renounces his sons, and preempts his daughters, but is eventually forgiven and joins the gods. The myth thus transcends Freudian connotations, and epitomizes many human vicissitudes and hopeful solutions.)

*Compulsion*: An act carried out (despite some conscious rejection and resistance by the patient) in accord with a persistent idea (*obsession*) and in order to avoid inexplicable *anxiety* should the impulse not be followed.

*Conation*: Covert motivation.

*Condensation*: A process by which many concepts may be represented by one. For instance, in symbolic imagery a snake may represent phallic erotism, slinking danger, low bestiality, pitiless aggressivity, mystic fascination, etc. So too, a *phobia* or a *conversion* symptom (q.v.) may condense and represent in compromise form many otherwise incompatible symbolizations and adaptations.

*Conditioning:* The process by which innate responses (*"unconditioned reflexes"*) when associated with new sensory stimuli, may thereafter be evoked by these stimuli (Chapter 10).

*Confabulation:* A tendency to substitute detailed but fantastic, inconsistent, and variable accounts—each version currently believed by the patient during its telling—to fill in gaps of memory produced by organic cerebral disease, e.g., as in *alcoholic* (*Korsakoff*) or *senile psychoses* (qq.v.).

*Conscience:* Conscious inhibitions through covert fear of punishment. *See* Guilt, Superego.

*Conversion:* In psychoanalytic theory, the process whereby sexual libido is "converted" and redirected into bodily (*autoplastic*) aberrations of behavior. The term is now mainly used to designate *hysterical* (q.v.) sensorimotor dysfunctions, such as blindness or paralysis (Briquet's syndrome, Appendix 1).

*Coprophilia (-phobia):* Attraction to (or excessive aversion to) feces or dirt.

*Countertransference:* 1. In psychoanalytic theory, the symbolic libidinal relationships, partly unconscious, of the analyst with the analytic patient (analysand) which may impair the ideal objectivity of the analytic process. 2. In general, the therapist's attitudes toward the patient, based on the former's interpersonal evaluations of the latter.

*Cretinism:* Congenital physical maldevelopment and mental retardation due to thyroid dysfunctions.

*Criminality:* Asocial, antisocial, or illegal conduct which is in accord with the conscious standards and intent of the individual. Theoretically, though not always practically, distinguishable (1) from *neurotic* or *sociopathic* behavior (qq.v.), in which the aberrant conduct is deviantly symbolic rather than indulged in for extrinsic gain, and (2) from *psychotic* behavior (q.v.), in which excesses of uncontrollable affect or distortions of generally accepted reality occasion the antisocial act.

*Cyclothymia:* A tendency to persistent, irrational, or exaggerated shifts in mood, especially with regard to alternations of euphoria (*hypomania, mania*) and depression (*hypothymia, melancholia*) (Chapter 4).

*Death Instinct:See* Instinct.

*Defense Mechanism:* 1. In psychoanalytic theory, a process by which the *Ego* (the orientative and integrative portion of the personality) partially satisfies the unconscious instinctive drives of the *Id* by behavior that conforms with the self-regulative demands of the *Superego* (qq.v.) 2. In general, adaptive modes of behavior constituting compromises among the needs of the organism and its experientially contingent perceptions and evaluations of its milieu (Chapter 8.).

*Déjà Vu:* An illusion of having experienced a new place or event previously.

*Delinquency:* Asocial, antisocial, illegal, or culturally nonconforming conduct in a minor.

*Delirium:* In modern usage, a state of disorientation and confusion (often with rapidly changing, generally fearful hallucinations) induced by the toxic effects of organic diseases or drugs (e.g. alcoholic *delirium tremens*).

*Delusion:* a fixed belief widely deviant from the cultural norm, and impervious to persuasion or reason.

*Dementia:* Deterioration of perceptive, integrative, and responsive (e.g. "intellectual") capacities due to organic disease of the brain.

*Dementia, Schizophrenic:* A term referring to the supposed "mental degeneration" in schizophrenia (q.v.). However, there is only disinterest in, and abandonment, disuse or distortion of, complex intellectual and social processes. Minimal deterioration of capacities (dementia) occurs unless secondary organic cerebral changes supervene as a result of drugs, the patient's physical debility or intercurrent diseases.

*Denial:* In psychoanalysis, an unconscious defense whereby the patient refuses to recognize or accept unwelcome conations or concepts.

*Depersonalization:* A subject's feeling or belief that he has lost his identity. D. is evanescent in *hypnagogic states* or in *neurotic* reactions, but may be persistent and accompanied by cosmic delusions in the *psychoses* (qq.v.).

*Depression:* A state characterized affectively by maintained dejection in mood, ideologically by gloomy ruminations or forebodings, and physiologically by the depressive syndrome (q.v.). Depressions range in intensity and persistence from evanescent "blues" to deep melancholia. *See* Psychoses, depressive.

*Depression, Reactive:* A self-limited state, the content, intensity, and duration of which have rational reference to "actual" rather than "symbolic" frustrations, deprivations, or adversities in the life of the patient. Distinguished from *psychosis* by the criteria listed under the latter (q.v.).

*Depression Syndrome:* Typically includes varying degrees of anorexia, loss of weight, constipation, or other gastrointestinal dysfunctions, easy fatigability and diminished sexual desire. In women, disturbances of menstruation are common; in men, relative impotence. Energy is generally decreased so that ideation and action are slowed, but diurnal variations (morning retardation, partially dispelled toward evening) may occur. However, there may be episodes of markedly increased appetite (bulimia), or a persistent, aimless, motor restlessness (agitation) may supervene (Chapter 4).

*Dereistic:*Unreal, delusional; i.e. not in accordance with generally accepted interpretations of space, time, and logic. Generally applied to schizophrenic or paranoid fantasies and their "irrational" organization.

*Desensitization:See* Reciprocal inhibition.

*Deterioration:* 1. Degeneration of intellectual capacities due to organic cerebral disease (e.g., *alcoholic* d; *senile* d.) as manifested by various *amnesias, aphasias, apraxias,* disturbances of category formation and impairment of energy (power factor), or loss of other intellectual functions.

*Diagnosis:* Comprehensive cognition of deviated vital processes and their somatic and behavioral effects. In modern psychiatry, diagnosis entails a balanced survey of the etiology, nature, context, and extent of all significant aberrations, as distinguished from mere superficial classification by "disease entities" (taxonomic nosology) (Chapter 4).

*Displacement:* The transfer of symbolic meaning and value from one object or concept to another: e.g., a mother may cherish a pet excessively after her child's death; a man may redirect unconscious hate of his father onto his boss; or a girl may compensate for genital guilt by obsessive-compulsive oral hygiene.

*Dissociation:* 1. The severance of normal relationships and sequences among motivations, thoughts, and affects. 2. Complex combinations of behavior patterns which, though integrated among themselves, may appear unrelated to the rest of the personality, giving rise to *"double"* or *"multiple personality"* (M. Prince) or to "encapsulated paranoia" (S. Rado).

*Distortion:* An adaptive alteration of a perception or concept to conform with the subject's wishes or prejudices; e.g., an aberrant apperception and evaluation of the characteristics of a loved or hated person or group.

*Down's Syndrome:* A genetic defect (trisomy 21) causing physical maldevelopment and intellectual retardation. Formerly *Mongolism.*

*Dream Function:* In psychoanalytic theory, a process by which dream fantasies express unconscious wishes and reexplore and allay anxieties through symbolic representation, resolution and interpretation.

*Economics:*1. In dynamic psychiatry, the study of the respective weighting, interaction, and balance of adaptive processes to produce final behavior. 2. In psychoanalytic theory, the distribution of *libido* according either to the pleasure principle, the psychosexual development or the *death instincts* (qq.v.).

*Ego:* In psychoanalytic theory, that portion or stratum of the "mind" or personality which is in contact with the environment through the senses, perceives and evaluates the milieu through intellectual functions, and directs behavior into acceptable compromises between the blind drives of the Id and the inhibitions (*conscience*) and idealizations (Ego-ideal) of the Superego (Chapter 8).

*Ego Analysis:* In psychoanalysis, the investigation of the methods (*defenses*) by which the Ego (a) resolves conflicts among Id drives or between these and excessive Superego inhibitions or goals, thus averting disruptive anxiety, and (b) adapts by "normal" or "neurotic" mechanisms to the demands of reality as analytically interpreted.

*Ego-Ideal:* In psychoanalytic theory, that portion or function of the Superego which orientates and directs the personality toward attainments—usually those of other persons with whom the subject has, in the past, identified his own interests.

*Eidetic Imagery:* Vivid, detailed, accurate, voluntarily controllable recall of previous sensory impressions, reported to be present in 60 percent of children and in some adults (Jaensch type).

*Electro-Convulsive Therapy:* A form of treating psychiatric disorders by passing an electric current through the brain, usually with the induction of convulsions and coma (Chapter 12).

*Emotion:* A state of affective excitation manifested during conative press or conflicts, and reflected in characteristic physiologic reactions and motor expressions (*e-moto*).

*Empathy:*The "objective" or "intellectual" recognition of the nature and significance of another's behavior, as distinguished from *sympathy*, derived from corresponding conative and affective experiences. *See* Rapport.

*Encephalitis:* Inflammation of the brain.

*Engram:*Neural repository of memory.

*Epicritic Sensitivity:* Accurate appreciation of light touch, temperature and point-to-point distance on the skin; distinguished from grosser *protopathic* sensations of pain or pressure (J. Head).

*Epilepsy:*A group of disorders characterized mainly by disturbances of conscious and motor convulsions often traceable by electroencephalography to cerebral dysrhythmias; generally episodic, except in the *continuous partial epilepsy* of Wilson and in *status epilepticus*. Distinguished from toxic convulsions and hysterical seizures in etiology, course, and prognosis (qq.v.) Cf. Epilepsy, major.

*Epilepsy, Jacksonian:* Recurrent convulsive movements beginning in one extremity and accompanied by minimal disturbances of consciousness. These may arise from circumscribed cerebral lesions (H. Jackson).

*Epilepsy, Major (Gran Mal):* Episodic disturbances or abolition of consciousness, with tonic contractions rapidly involving the whole body (*ophishotonos*), followed by violent clonic movements, during which there may be urinary or fecal incontinence. The attack may be heralded by a prodromal *aura* (sensory, affective, or hallucinatory experiences) and the convulsions may be immediately preceded by an explosive ("Hippocratic") *epileptic cry*. If the patient is not prepared for the seizure he generally falls, and may bite his tongue or injure himself during the convulsions. *Postdromata* often consist of lassitude, muscular weakness or soreness, headaches, and amnesia for the seizure. Epilepsy may be distinguished from toxic convulsive states (e.g., strychnine tetany) and *hysterical seizures* (qq.v.) by its etiology, symptoms, and course.

*Epilepsy, Minor (Petit Mal):* Characterized by relatively mild muscular movements, or sometimes only by momentary impairments of consciousness (absences), during which, the patient may automatically continue his previous activity (minor *fugue*).

*Epileptic Equivalents:* Any episodic sensory, motor, or experiential phenomena that may replace convulsive seizures in epilepsy (psychic epilepsy).

*Epilelptic Fugue:* A state of disturbed, clouded, bewildered, or dreamlike consciousness with integrated but automatic and occasionally violent activity following epileptic seizures. The fugue may persist from minutes to (in rare cases) days, and is thereafter generally submerged in almost complete amnesia.

*Epileptic Status (status epilepticus):* Incessant or nearly continuous epileptic seizures which, in extreme cases, may lead to exhaustion and death if not therapeutically controlled.

*Epileptoid Personality:* Thought by some to comprise traits of intense affective ambivalence, obsessive-compulsive tendencies, hypersensitivity, mysticism and religiosity, and propensity for vacillating instability between extremes of impulsive behavior. However, it is probable that the concept of an "epileptic character type" has no independent validity, and in the relatively few patients in whom such traits are marked, they represent secondary neurotic reactions to the epileptic disorder rather than a correlated constitutional deviation.

*Epinosic (Secondary) Gain: Paranosic* advantages derived from an illness or behavior disorder, as distinguished from the essential determinants and phenomena of the illness itself.

*Existentialism*:Phenomenologic knowledge of and responsibility for "the self" (Chapter 9).

*Extinction*:The disappearance of a *conditioned reflex* (Pavlov) when it is repeatedly elicited without reinforcement by the *unconditioned reflex* through the provision of a reward (Chapter 10).

*Extrasensory Perception (ESP)*: Information supposedly acquired other than by the five acknowledged sensory routes.

*Extroversion*: Interest and participation in the "external" world, as distinguished from *intraversion*, or preoccupation with endogenous "self-centered" fantasies and autistic behavior (C. Jung).

*Euphoria*:Illusory sense of excessive well-being.

*Fetish*:A symbolically cherished object.

*Fixation*:1. The persistence of a definite goal or pattern of behavior. 2. In psychoanalytic theory, the continuation into later life of some *pregenital* (e.g., *oral* or *anal*) phase of interest in, or evaluation of, objects (*libidinal cathexis*, qq.v.).

*Formication*:Sensation of crawlings on the skin.

*Fugue*:A state in which the patient's consciousness and behavior, though they may be well integrated, show an apparent break in continuity with previous patterns. *Epileptic fugues* (q.v.) leave an almost complete *amnesia* for their duration; *hysterical* fugues leave a lacunar and generally penetrable amnesia (qq.v.).

*Galvanic Skin Response (GSR):* Decreased dermal resistance to a direct current during emotional excitement.

*Ganser Syndrome*:Pretended insanity.

*Gender Identity*:Cultural adoption of a gender role, as opposed to *genetic sexuality*.

*General Paresis (dementia paralytica)*: A behavior disorder, the organic precipitating cause of which is syphilitic infection of the brain; in late cases, a frank psychosis characterized by *dementia*, dysarthria, and habit deterioration. Pathognomonic neurologic signs may appear and dominate the clinical picture.

*Genotype*: *See* phenotype.

*Gestalt*: Holistic integration of perceptions and responses. *See also* Psychology, Gestalt.

*Grandiosity*: Delusions of being wealthy, famous, powerful, omniscient, etc.

*Guilt*: Dread of loss of love or retributive punishment for impulses or deeds forbidden in earlier experiences.

*Hallucination*: An auditory, visual, tactile (*haptic*), or other perception accepted as real by the subject but occasioned by no apparent external sensory stimuli. Hallucinations differ from *hypnagogic* (q.v.) or dream imagery in that no corrective reorientation occurs immediately after the imagery ceases, or on waking, although the rapidly changing, fearful hallucinations of toxic *deliria* may be recalled as unreal after recovery.

*Hermaphrodite*: Anatomically bisexual.

*Homeostasis*: The tendency of organisms to maintain their metabolic processes insofar as possible within optimal limits for individual and race survival (C. Bernard, W. Cannon).

*Hypnagogic*: Semiconscious state, usually preceding sleep.

*Hypnocatharsis*: *See* Catharsis.

*Hypnosis (Hypnotism)*: A passive state usually produced by monotonous, reiterated suggestion of relaxation, sleep, and control by the hypnotist, in which the subject shows increased amenability and responsiveness to directions or commands, provided that these do not conflict seriously with the subject's own conscious or covert wishes. "Forgotten" memories may be recalled, and altered states of sensibility, perception, or motor function may be induced. Acceptable acts may also be compulsively performed by the subject after the hypnotic *trance* has been terminated (*posthypnotic suggestion*), and the patient may profess a directed forgetfulness for his experiences during the trance (*posthypnotic amnesia*) (Chapter 8).

*Hysteria (Briquet's Syndrome):* 1. A state of neurotic sensorimotor dysfunction, e.g., pseudo-blindness, paralysis, or convulsions. 2. The lay term for great emotional and motor excitation ("hysterics") should not be used in this sense in psychiatric description or diagnosis.

*Id:* In psychoanalytic theory, a general term for all unconsciously determined instincts or libidinal strivings (q.v.), constituting the conative "portion" of the psyche (Chapter 8).

*Identification:* Wishful adoption, mainly unconscious, of the personality characteristics or identity of another individual, generally one possessing advantages which the subject envies and desires.

*Identity Crisis:* Intense doubt as to one's role in life.

*Idiocy, Moral (Moral Insanity of Prichard):* Almost obsolete terms connoting a serious lack of "moral sense" or "moral development," i.e., the inadequate establishment of social responsibilities and adaptations. *Cf.* Criminality, Sociopathy.

*Illusion:* Misinterpretation of a sensory percept; usually fleeting or correctable by closer or supplementary examination of the stimulus which induced the illusion.

*Imbecility:* An outmoded term indicating general intellectual deficiency such that the average intelligence level is between about one-quarter and one-half normal. Imbeciles nearly always require institutional care.

*Inhibition*:1. In general, the internal checking or restraint of a conation, affect, thought, or act. 2. In psychoanalytic theory, the prevention of Id instincts from reaching conscious recognition and response, because of specific Ego controls directed by the Superego (qq.v.). 3. In reflexology (a) the submergence of a positive or *excitatory conditioned reflex* by a contrary *inhibitory* one, (b) the supposed occurrence of a radiating inhibitory process over the cerebral cortex, controlling the corresponding neural reflex arcs.

*Insanity*:A vague legal term variously connoting inability "to distinguish right from wrong," or a "mental state in which the patient is unable to care for himself or constitutes a danger to others." To be distinguished from the psychiatric concept of psychosis (q.v.).

*Insight*:1. Clinically, the patient's own explanation of his illness, progressively judged "distorted," "incomplete," "good," etc., by the observer insofar as it coincides with his own theoretic formulations. 2. In psychoanalysis, the extent of a patient's true (as opposed to merely professed or verbal) understanding of the origins and unconscious dynamisms of his behavior. 3. In Gestalt psychology, the phenomenon of sudden grasp (*ah ha! erlebnis*) of a perceptual configuration or of the solution to a problem.

*Instinct*:1. A conative psychologic term with variable meaning, but generally connoting an inborn tendency toward specific patterns of behavior (e.g., the sex instinct, the exploratory instinct, etc.) 2. In older psychoanalytic theory, a primary tendency toward life and reproduction (Eros) or toward destruction, dissolution, and death (Thanatos).

*Intelligence*:The sum total and degree of development of the organism's capacities to perceive, differentiate, integrate, and manipulate its environment (C. Tolman). C. Spearman contends that there is an overall index (g) of *general intelligence,* plus factors for perseveration (p), fluency (f), will (w), and speed (s). Others divide intelligence into less interdependent capacities:

e.g., *abstract i., mechanical i.,* and *social i.* (E. Thorndike), or various special (statistically determined) vectors of intellectual capacity such as *memory (m), verbal fluency* (w), *space visualization (s), number facility (n),* and, possibly, other factors of induction, deduction, speed of reaction time, perception, judgment, *closure* (including flexibility), and rate of reversal of ambiguous perceptions (L. Thurstone). In any case, the ordinary tests (q.v.) of *general intelligence* (e.g., the Stanford-Binet or Kuhlman) indicate only rough averages of these abilities; moreover, they often do not take adequate account of intercurrent conative and affective factors, or of the previous training and experiences of the subject.

*Intelligence Quotient (I.Q.):* A figure indicating the subject's performance on some test of intelligence (q.v.) in relation to the statistical norm for his age; e.g., a child of twelve (*chronological age*) whose performance stopped at the eight and a half year level would have an I.Q. of 71. *See* Intelligence.

*Introject:* In psychoanalysis, the imaginal incorporation of significant figures into the Id or Ego variously regarded as favorable or deleterious (e.g., the "good" or "bad" mother) (Chapter 8).

*Introversion:* Preoccupation with self.

*Intuition:* A sudden understanding or conviction not reached by conscious reasoning; usually an integration of stored data and wishes which reach consciousness as an illuminating "insight" or inspiration. The resulting behavior may or may not be adaptive or favorable.

*Korsakoff Psychosis:* A toxic psychosis (usually alcoholic) characterized by inflammatory or retrogressive changes in peripheral nerves (polyneuritis), disorientations, amnesia with *confabulation* and intellectual deterioration (*dementia*) (qq.v.).

*Latency Period:* In psychoanalysis, libidinal quiescence between the oedipal ages of four or five and puberty (Chapter 9).

*Libido*: 1. In psychoanalytic theory, the energy associated with the instincts of the Id. 2. In a more limited sense (medical and lay) the desire for sexual relationships; sex drive.

*Love*: 1. an affect or sentiment evoked by a person (concept or object) that fulfills one's needs or expectations. (This definition is not recommended for domestic use.) 2. "Love is the effort of two solitudes to protect and touch and greet each other" — Rainer Marie Rilke. *See* Rapport.

*Malingering*: The deliberate simulation of disease; usually, however, by neurotic individuals.

*Mania*: A syndrome of excessive elation, ideation, distractibility and restless activity. *See* Psychosis, manic.

*Manifest Content*: Recalled events in dreams, interpreted psychoanalytically as *latent content*. *See* Dreams (Chapter 8).

*Mannerism*: A characteristic expression, gesture, or movement. When stereotyped and unconsciously repetitious, but minor, it is termed a *tic*. Such movements may become symbolically bizarre and persistent in schisophrenia (q.v.).

*Masculine Protest*: Overassertion of virility or dominance in either sex (A. Adler).

*Masochism*: 1. In sexology, erotic pleasure derived from physical pain. 2. In older psychoanalytic theory, the satisfaction of destructive instincts (Thanatos) "turned against the self." 3. In Biodynamics, the satisfaction of bodily needs through learned adaptive patterns, certain aspects of which may appear unpleasant or painful to an observer.

*Mechanism*: 1. In psychoanalytic theory, the interaction among psychic "structures": e.g., the Ego "defends itself" against the Id by the "mechanism" of repression (qq.v.). 2. In Biodynamics, a process of contingent and total organismic adaptation devoid of any implication of isolated patterns.

*Melancholia:*A severe depressive psychosis (q.v.).

*Mental Hygiene:*A term employed by A. Meyer to designate the development of optimal modes of personal and social conduct and the prevention of psychiatric disorders.

*Mesmerism:*"Animal magnetism" of Mesmer; later *hypnosis* (Chapter 8).

*Metapsychology:*A behavioral theory that cannot be verified or disproved by observation or reasoning.

*Migraine:*A disorder characterized by recurrent attacks of severe localized or one-sided (*hemicranial*) headaches, which are often preceded or accompanied by visual disturbances, gastrointestinal dysfunctions, and physical fatigue or prostration.

*Mind*: 1. A reification of the dynamics comprising a person's motivations, affects, intelligence, values, beliefs, etc. 2. Operationally, the phenomena of body in internal (including speech) and external action (Chapter 1).

*M'Naughten Rule*: A legal precedent from the murder trial of Daniel M'Naughten (England, 1843) to the effect (a) that "any act committed by an idiot, imbecile, or lunatic" cannot be adjudged a crime, and (b) that such persons cannot be tried and punished by criminal procedures if it can be shown that they were aware neither of the "nature" of their act, nor that it was "wrong." This precedent is incorporated into the criminal law of most of our states.

*Moron:*1. A mentally defective person, with average intelligence (IQ) of 50 (*low grade m.*) to 79 (*high grade m.*) as estimated by standard intelligence tests with a "norm" of about a hundred. 2. A lay or journalistic term incorrectly applied to sexual perverts.

*Mourning:*A state of grief and sadness over a loss; theoretically distinguished from *depression* or *melancholia* (q.v.) by the absence of marked self-recriminations, persistent agitation, a severe depressive syndrome or suicidal impulses. *Cf.* Psychoses, depressive.

*Multiple Personality:*One or more disparate roles successively acted out by one individual (M. Prince).

*Narcissism or Narcism:*From Narcissus, who, for rejecting his mistress, Echo, was condemned by Nemesis to fall in love with his own reflected image. In psychoanalysis, equivalent to original self-love, or to the reidentification with, or fantasied *reincorporation* of, objects or persons given a temporary investiture (*cathexis*) of object-love. The first form is called *primary narcissism*, the rederived form *secondary narcissism*.

*Narcoanalysis:See* Catharsis.

*Narcolepsy:*Recurrent episodes of trancelike or sleep states, occurring with no or little warning, and persisting from a few seconds to several hours. They may be of neurotic etiology. *See* epileptic equivalents.

*Narcosynthesis:* A therapeutic procedure in which the patient is given a hypnotic drug (e.g., Pentothal) to alleviate his acute anxiety, permitted to express his repressed memories, affects and conflicts (cf. *Catharsis*) and then guided by the therapist to conative and emotional reintegration, behavioral readjustments, and social rehabilitation (J. Spiegel).

*Need:* A psychophysiologic (metabolic) deficiency or imbalance translated dynamically into behavior (characterized variously as motivated by desires, drives, goals, instincts, wishes, strivings, etc.) intended for the direct or indirect satisfaction of the deficiency.

*Negativism:*Excessive opposition to directives.

*Neologism:*An individually coined, usually incomprehensible word.

*Nerves, Nervous, Nervous Breakdown, Nervous Spells, etc.*: Lay euphemisms used vaguely to describe behavior disorders. Such terms should not be used, other than in quotes from the patient, in psychiatric description or diagnosis.

*Neurasthenia*: A euphemistic term for a vague group of symptoms consisting of muscular weakness or fatigability, inertia, petulant irritability, aversion to effort, variable aches and pains, and minor organic dysfunctions. At present the term has no connotation of organic disease of the nervous system.

*Neuroses*: A group of behavior disorders representing suboptimal adaptations to biodynamic stresses, conflicts, or uncertainties. Neuroses are characterized symptomatically by 1. *anxiety*, with its recurrent physiologic manifestations (*see Anxiety syndrome*), or 2. by various sensorimotor (*hysterical*) or organic-neurotic (*psychosomatic*) dysfunctions (qq.v.). Generally, the history reveals previous sensitivities and maladaptations to frustration and conflict, exacerbation of somatic symptomatology under duress, and partial recovery when stress is relieved either spontaneously or under therapy. For theoretic and practical purposes, neuroses are distinguished from psychoses by the criteria listed under the latter (q.v.), although all forms of transition occur (Chapter 4).

*Neurosis, Conversion*: A neurosis (q.v.) characterized predominantly by dysfunctions of (a) sensation or motility (*hysteria*) or (b) one or more organ-systems (organ neuroses). Frank anxiety or *obsessive-compulsive* features (q.v.) may be minimal, especially when the hysterical symptoms serve as adequate adaptations.

*Neurosis, Obsessive-Compulsive*: A neurosis characterized predominantly by admittedly irrational but persistent thoughts and impulses, usually combined with phobias. When these are resisted or transgressed, an acute *anxiety syndrome* occurs (qq.v.).

*Nirvana Fantasy*: From Buddhist theology, a state in which there is no desire, no affect, and no strife—only pervasive peace. Differs from uterine fantasies (q.v.) in that the latter may connote deeply regressive tendencies.

*Obsession:*A persistent, conscious desire or idea, recognized as being more or less irrational by the subject, which usually impels compulsive acts on pain of *anxiety* (qq.v.) if they are not performed. Obsessions can often be analyzed as conscious reflections of conflictual wishes.

*Occupational Therapy:*Treatment by diverting the patient's energies into constructive recreational or manual pursuits satisfactory to him.

*Oligophrenia:*Mental retardation (a. Meyer).

*Onanism:*Coitus interruptus.

*Orgasm:*The height of erotic pleasure, just preceding detumescence and relaxation. Generally refers to erotic sensations centered in the genitals, but orgastic sensations in the mouth, breast, anus, or even skin (as in masturbatory-equivalent scratching) have been described.

*Orientation:* Awareness of place, time, circumstances, and interpersonal relationships.

*Orthopsychiatry:*The comprehensive, interdisciplinary study of the phenomena and dynamisms of the development of "normal" behavior, with emphasis on child and preventive psychiatry and *"mental hygiene"* (q.v.).

*Overcompensation:* 1. An adaptive process particularly stressed by Alfred Adler, whereby a person overreacts to initial deficiencies, handicaps, or inhibitions in some sphere of activity by becoming exceedingly adept in that field (e.g., Demosthenes, afflicted with an impediment of speech in his youth, strove for, and succeeded in reaching the pinnacles of oratorical power). 2. In psychoanalytic theory, an excessive overplay of any defense mechanisms; e.g., revealing overpolitness toward a disliked person; or compulsive *satyriasis* (q.v.) as a defense against covert homosexual tendencies.

*Overdetermination*:A process whereby a single behavior pattern becomes adaptive to many covert needs, thus rendering it particularly fixed and resistant to therapy. For instance, a *hysterical paralysis* (q.v.) of an arm may be a combat flier's initial reaction to a crash landing, but later the same symptom may also come to symbolize (a) a denial of his own mobilized aggressions, (b) a rationalized excuse for not returning to a hated civilian job, (c) expiation for a regressive dependence on a government pension, etc. In this sense, overdetermination parallels the process of *condensation* (q.v.) in the formation of verbal and dream symbols.

*Panic*:Extreme anxiety, with blind flight or marked disorganization of behavior.

*Paralysis Agitans (Parkinson's Disease)*: An organic disease of the brain, particularly of the basilar nuclei, caused by inflammation (*encephalitis*), drugs, or senile changes, and characterized by progressive muscular dystonia, spasticity, and tremor, disturbances in motor control (*festination, retropulsion,* and *akasthesia*) and sometimes by outbreaks of irrational rage and excitement.

*Paranoia*:Delusions of gradiosity or persecution. *See* Psychoses.

*Parapsychology*:A system based on postulates of *extrasensory perception* (q.v.).

*Parasympathetic Nervous System*: The cranio-sacral, vagal, cholinergic and generally anabolic and inhibitory portion of the sympathetic nervous system (q.v.).

*Paresis*:An organic psychosis (q.v.) caused by syphilis of the brain, and generally characterized by affective instability with recurrent excitements, muscular tremors, speech disturbances, pathognomonic changes in the pupillary reactions and in the spinal fluid, and progressive behavioral deterioration. (General paresis).

*Paresthesia*:Deviant tactile sensation.

*Pavor Nocturnus*:Nightmares or night terrors.

*Pederasty*:Anal intercourse with children.

*Pedophilia*:Sexual attraction to children.

*Perception*:The integration of sensory stimuli to form an image, the configuration and interpretation of which is influenced by past experiences.

*Perseveration*:Irrational repetitions of ideas or acts.

*Persona* One's external facade, distinguished from his internal *anima* or *animus* (C. Jung).

*Personality*:Comprises the sum total of the unique behavior patterns of an individual, particularly those concerned in his social relationships (*cf*. Chapter 6).

*Persuasion*: A form of therapeutic influence, usually conceived as verbal, by which the patient's motivations, covert as well as conscious, are directed toward goals desired by the therapist.

*Phenomenology*:"Reality" as interpreted by the self rather than as an absolute.

*Phenotype*:Physical build, as the milieu and individual experiences influence the inherited *genotype*.

*Phobia*:A morbid aversion to an object, situation or act, generally derived from its symbolic reference to an anxiety-ridden previous experience or series of experiences.

*Phrenology:*Correlation of personality traits with conformation of the skull (F. Gall). A concept now discarded.

*Pica:*Perversion of the appetite; toxic feeding.

*Placebo:*Object or maneuver used solely to placate another.

*Pleasure Principle:* In psychoanalytic theory, the seeking of release from libidinal tensions (giving pleasure) as distinguished from various manifestations of the death-instinct or Thanatos (such as in the *repetition compulsion* or *masochism,* qq.v.).

*Preconscious:*Recallable concepts.

*Prejudice:*An intellectual set which covertly biases or distorts a subject's apperception and evaluation of later experiences according to predetermined attitudes.

*Prevention in Psychiatry:Primary,* to forestall behavior disorders genetically or environmentally. *Secondary:* To limit their occurrence. *Tertiary:* To treat them. Obviously, these "preventive" rubrics overlap.

*Primary Process:* In psychoanalysis, instinctive, unreasoned conations, thoughts or actions. *See* Id (Chapter 9).

*Privileged Communication:* Information that ethically cannot be revealed by a physician.

*Projection:* An unconscious defense process whereby the subject attributes his own motivations, concepts, or acts to others.

*Prolonged Sleep:*Treatment of behavior disorders by continuous sleep (1–20 days) induced by drugs such as paraldehyde or Amytal (*Dauerschlaf*).

*Psychoanalysis:* A psychologic system of research, theory, and therapy the broad outlines of which were propounded by Sigmund Freud (1856-1939). (Chapter 8).

*Psychobiology:* An eclectic system of behavior research, theory, and therapy outlined by Adolf Meyer (1866-1944). *See* Reaction Types and index.

*Psychodrama:* Group therapy in which patients or therapists act out roles relevant to each others' lives (J. Moreno).

*Psychology, Gestalt:* A psychological system (Wertheimer, Koffka, Kohler, et al.) which rejects elemental stimulus-response *(reflex)* concepts, stresses the indivisible wholeness of perceptual configurations *(Gestalten)*, and emphasizes the sudden "insightful" nature of learning as opposed to trial-and-error or automatic "association" (Chapter 11).

*Psychoneuroses:* A term now generally used as equivalent to *neurosis* (q.v.) or sometimes as implying severe neuroses with larval or minimal psychotic tendencies or admixtures.

*Psychoses:* A group of grave disorders of behavior, most of which satisfy the legal criteria of "insanity" in that the patient is unable to care for himself and/or constitutes a danger to others. Psychoses, however, also fulfill one or more of the following psychiatric criteria; (1) Loss of contact with, or marked distortion of socially accepted interpretations of reality (as shown in deviated perceptions, thinking disorders, *hallucinations,* or *delusions*). (2) Severe and persistent disorders of *affect* (e.g., manic *euphoria,* depressive *melancholia,* or *schizophrenic* emotional blunting, and lack of correspondence between affect and idea). (3) Marked *regression,* with (a) retreat from, or perversion of, social relationships (e.g., perverse passivity, dependency, or aggressivity), or (b) habit reversions (e.g., open masturbation, soiling, etc.). (4) Personality disintegration, so that elementary erotic and hostile impulses or *automatisms* are released from control. (5) (a) Acute derangement of perceptive-interpretative-manipulative *(intellectual)* capacities (as in toxic *deliria*), or (b) the permanent deterioration of such capacities (as in psychoses with organic cerebral disease).

*Psychoses, Depressive*: Variously characterized by melancholic fixation of mood, retardation of apperception and response, self-depreciatory preoccupations (ideas of inadequacy, of guilt, and of being hated), morbid preoccupation with anticipated punishment, nihilistic fantasies ("all is hopeless," or "lost"), episodes of agitation, petulant demanding helplessness and regression, suicidal tendencies, and a marked depressive *physiologic syndrome* comprising insomnia, anorexia, loss of weight, sexual disturbances, and various organic (especially gastrointestinal) dysfunctions.

*Psychoses, Involutional*: Originally considered to be a definite syndrome characterized mainly by melancholia and agitation, generally progressing to hebetude and intellectual deterioration. Actually, psychoses occurring in the involutional period vary widely in etiology, clinical expression, and prognosis (Chapter 3, 4, and 15).

*Psychoses, Manic*: Characterized by extreme emotional lability (though with superficially euphoric affect), psychomotor hyperactivity (uninhibited flow of free-associative speech and conduct), hypersensitivity to stimuli with marked distractibility, and a tendency to unorganized delusions of grandiosity. Manic episodes are generally self-limited in duration; occasionally, they are apt to recur regularly (*cyclic manic*) or in alternation with periods of depression (*manic-depressive psychosis*). Rare cases of *chronic mania* (J. Schoat) have been reported.

*Psychoses, Organic*: Severe disorders of behavior in which pathologic changes in the body, especially in the central nervous system, are etiologically significant (Chapters 4 and 13).

*Psychoses, Paranoiac*: Relatively rare (about 4 percent incidence) and characterized by well-systematized, slowly progressive delusions of influence, reference or persecution which, although based on false premises and interpretations, are relatively logical and consistent, and accompanied by appropriate affect. Paranoia is distinguished from the *affective psychoses* and from *schizophrenia* by minimal affective distortion or personality disintegration. (*see* Schizophrenia, paranoid).

*Psychoses, Senile:*Caused by degenerative or arteriosclerotic changes in the brain, and generally characterized by progressive dementia (aphasic defects, amnesia for recent events), habit deteriorations (e.g., loss of cultural interests, garrulity, hoarding, personal uncleanliness) and regressions to puerile affectivity (e.g., the petulant dependence and selfishness of "second childhood"). *See* Pick's and Alzheimer's disease (Chapter 4).

*Psychosomatic Medicine:*The study, theory, and application of the dynamics of total behavior (biodynamics) in relation to the practice of medicine and its several specialties.

*Psychotherapy:*The science and art of influencing behavior so as to make it (a) more efficient and satisfactory to the individual and (b) more compatible with social norms.

*Rapport:*Empathy and trust between individuals; in psychiatry, between patient and therapist.

*Rationalization:* The conscious justification (usually on grounds of "reason," "logic," or social expediency) of attitudes, concepts, and acts after these have already been determined by covert or conscious motivations.

*Reaction Formation:* In psychoanalytic theory, the process whereby conscious wishes, affects, ideations, or modes of conduct are made defensively contrary to rejected impulses; e.g., a father's overtly reactive cruelty to a daughter to whom he is incestuously attracted.

*Reaction Type:* In *psychobiology* (A. Meyer), the predominant behavior pattern or *ergasia* of a psychiatric patient: i.e., *anergasia* (intellectually defective), *dysergasia* (toxic), *pathergasia* (organic), *holergasia* (psychotic), *meregasia* (neurotic part-reaction), *oliger-*

*gasia* (retarded), *parergasia* (schizophrenic) and *thymergasia* (affective psychoses).

*Reality Principle:* In psychoanalytic theory, the modification of the expression of unconscious libidinal drives (*pleasure principle, Eros*) or of the death instincts (*Thanatos* or the *Nirvana* principle) by rational consideration of the requirements of "reality."

*Reciprocal Inhibition:* In behavior therapy (J. Wolpe), the mitigation of aversions by increasingly pleasant reassociations.

*Reference, Delusion of:* A fixed, irrational belief that one is the object of the thoughts and actions of others.

*Reflex:* In neurophysiology, a sensimotor neural pathway. *Cf.* Conditioning and the Index for other connotations of the term.

*Regression:* 1. The resumption, under stress, of earlier and experientially more satisfactory modes of behavior. 2. In psychoanalytic theory, the return to infantile phases of libidinal organization; i.e., *narcissistic, oral* or *anal* (qq.v.).

*REM Sleep:* Dreaming sleep accompanied by rapid eye movements; occurs about a fifth of total sleep time.

*Repetition Compulsion:* Drive to reenact traumatic experiences (S. Freud).

*Repression:* The automatic and unconsciously defensive process of banishing dangerous desires, affects or ideas, singly or together, from awareness; distinguished from suppression, in which the control exercised is seemingly deliberate and conscious.

*Resistance:* In psychiatric, and especially psychoanalytic, therapy, the reluctance of the patient to relinquish accustomed patterns of thinking, feeling, and acting, however deviant, in favor of new and untried modes of adaptation. In psychonalytic theory, resistance often has the more limited meaning of the Ego's refusal to accept insight into the Unconscious, as shown by the patient's covert rejection of interpretation or the development of a *negative transference* (qq.v.).

*Satyriasis:*Exaggerated, diffuse sexual activity in a male.

*Schizophrenia:* A group of variable psychotic (q.v.) syndromes characterized predominantly by: 1. General blunting and distortion of *affect,* especially in relation to professed ideational content and interpersonal relationships. 2. Bizarre perceptual and category formations and thinking disturbances, loosely organized into fantastic *delusional systems,* and sometimes projected as *hallucinatory experiences.* 3. *Regression* to primitive forms of *narcissistic,* erotic, or aggressive expression. 4. Disintegration of behavior with the appearance of *stereotypes* and motor *automatisms* (qq.v.). For the various clinical forms of schizophrenia, *see* Chapter 4).

*Schizophrenia, Catatonic :* Characterized by motor disturbances (*catalepsy, flexibilitas cerea, negativism, mannerisms*), stupors, or acute outbreaks of hallucinatory excitement, and occasional periods of remission.

*Schizophrenia, Hebephrenic:* A highly variable form characterized by early onset, insidious distortion and blunting of affect, inconstant *hallucinosis,* and fragmentary *delusional formations,* the development of symbolic mannerisms and *stereotypes,* and progressive deterioration of personal and social habits (K. Kahlbaum, E. Kraepelin).

*Schizophrenia, Latent :* Schizoid or schizophrenic tendencies likely to find overt expression under unfavorable stress.

*Schizophrenia, Paranoid :* A form in which delusions of *reference* and influence are prominent; distinguished from *paranoia* in that (a) the delusions are highly fantastic, logically bizarre, and poorly systematized, and (b) other schizophrenic criteria (affect distortion, pervasive behavioral disintegration, etc.) are also present. *See* Psychoses, paranoiac.

*Schizophrenia, Process:* A term sometimes used to designate schizophrenic "dementia" in which organic changes in the brain are found (or are postulated to be) important etiologic factors.

*Schizophrenia, Pseudoneurotic* : Ambulatory schizophrenia underlying severe hysterical, somatic, obsessive-compulsive-phobic, or character neuroses (P. Hoch, S. Rado).

*Schizophrenic Deterioration:* Disintegration of habit patterns and disuse of intellectual capacities consequent on schizophrenic contraction of interests and deviations or perversions of behavior; however, except in so-called *process* (organic) schizophrenia, there is no demonstrable loss of basic abilities.

*Screen Memory:* 1. A relatively acceptable memory recalled in place of one charged (*cathected*) with greater anxiety. 2. A retrospective illusion.

*Secondary Gains:* Incidental (*epinosic*) advantages of a neurosis.

*Secondary Process:* Rationally adaptive (*Ego-syntonic*) as opposed to unreasoned instinctive (Id) thought and conduct.

*Shock Treatment:* The subjection of psychiatric patients to convulsive doses of Metrazol, carbon dioxide, insulin or Indoklon, or to an electric current passed through the brain (Chapter 12).

*Sociopath, Sociopathic Personality:* Generally refers to an individual who is not readily classifiable as predominantly intellectually defective, autoplastically neurotic, or definitely psychotic (qq.v.), but whose behavior is characterized by episodic impulsivity, irresponsibility, lack of emotional control, and inadequate or unstable educational, marital, occupational, and other social adaptations. Sociopaths are prone to come into conflict with police or other social authorities—a tendency used by some to distinguish them from a group of "neurotic characters" who keep their eccentricities and aberrations (e.g., extreme prejudices, excessive religiosity, obsessive-compulsive-phobic behavior, etc.)

within the bounds of law and custom. Formerly *psychopathic personality.*

*Sodomy:* Anal intercourse.

*Stereotypy:* Repetitiousness in speech or action.

*Sublimation:* A "normal" process of directing unconscious and essentially selfish motivations into socially acceptable services or creative activities.

*Substitution:* The replacement of conations, affects, concepts or acts by others with a lesser charge of anxiety.

*Suggestion:* A process of gestural or verbal communication by which one person may use another's evaluations of him (*transference relations,* q.v.) to channelize the latter's behavior into desired patterns.

*Superego:* In psychoanalytic theory, that portion or function of the psyche which (a) as *conscience,* prohibits the Ego from direct forms of instinct-expression and thereby prompts the individual to utilize various *defense mechanisms* against unconscious Id impulses, and (b) as Ego-ideal, channels behavior along patterns similar to those of other individuals with whom the subject wishes to identify (i.e., whose advntages he covertly or consciously desires) (Chapter 8).

*Suppression:* The deliberate subjugation and control of impulses, ideas, affects, and acts felt to be dangerous.

*Surrogate:* One person placed in another's role.

*Symbiosis:* An intense, mutually advantageous relationship between or among organisms.

*Symbol:* The more or less remotely displaced representation of an experience in imagery.

*Sympathetic Nervous System:* That portion of the nervous system that innervates the organs and glands of the body, as distinguished from the peripheral nerves which innervate the muscles and sense organs. The SNS is usually divided functionally into the *orthosympathetic* NS (generally catabolic) and the *parasympathetic* NS (generally anabolic) (qq.v.).

*T-Groups:* Unstructured communication to establish "self-realization" and empathy among small assemblages of individuals for purposes of training (T) or "sensitivity."

*Therapy:*In psychiatry, the science, techniques and art of exerting a favorable influence on behavior disorders by every ethical means available.

*Transactional Analysis:*Clarification of personal interactions in terms of "child," "parent," and "adult," with analysis of individual "scripts," maneuvers for advantage, etc. (E. Berne) (Chapter 11).

*Transference:*1. In general, the attribution (transfer) of desires, feelings, and relationships, originally experienced by the subject with regard to his parents and siblings, onto other persons who, in the subject's residual attitudes, are assigned supportive, authoritative, competitive or other roles in his later life. 2. More specifically in psychoanalysis the unconscious attitude of the patient toward the analyst and the role in which the latter is fantasied, e.g., maternal, rivalrous, submissive, erotic, etc.

*Transsexualism:*A desire to be changed physically to the opposite sex and to act accordingly.

*Transvestism:*Pleasure in dressing as the opposite sex.

*Triage:*In clinical psychiatry, the rapid diagnosis and therapy of acute behavior disorders in crisis situations.

*Types of Character, Personality, or Physique:*The various classifications are legion, but the following are most often referred to in the literature:

*Draper, G.* The hereditary characteristics of an individual (*biotype* as derived from *genotype*), further modified by environment (*phenotype*);
*Galenic-Hippocratic* (humoral). CHOLERIC (dominated by "yellow bile"): mercurial, irritable, impulsive. MELANCHOLIC (dominated by "black bile"): brooding, emotional, depressive. PHLEGMATIC (dominated by "phlegm"): slow, apathetic, stolid. SANGUINE (dominated by "strong blood"): impulsive, active, optimistic.
*Hippocratic.* HABITUS APOPLECTICUS. Thick-set, heavy body-build, susceptible to apoplexy. HABITUS PHYSICUS. Tall, slender, angular body-build, susceptible to pulmonary disease.
*Jung C.* INTRAVERTED. Self-concerned, ruminative, remote, imaginative, inclined to schizoid behavior. EXTROVERTED. Objective, sensitive to external affairs, emotionally labile, active, energetic, inclined to manic-depressive disorders. Jung also speaks of: FEELING TYPES, with labile and sensitive affect, and INTUITIVE TYPES markedly influenced by their unconscious racial and personal heritage.
*Kretschmer, E.* ASTHENIC OR LEPTOSOMIC. Characterized by leanness, underweight, flat chest, and underdeveloped muscular system, especially marked in the *phthisoid* subgroup. ATHLETIC.Characterized by robust musculo-skeletal development. DYSPLASTIC.A group of "body-types" which show wide anthropometric deviations from the other three types, and which tend to *schizothymia.* PYKNIC.Short, stocky, large body cavities, bradycephalic; inclined to *cyclothymia.*
*Sheldon, W.* ECTOMORPHIC. Characterized by predominant development of the embryonic ectoderm (epidermis, sense organs, and central nervous system), hence sensitive and hyperreactive. ENDOMORPHIC. Predominant endoderm derivatives (mainly gastrointestinal organic), hence interest in nutritive living. MESOMORPHIC. Predominantly skeletal and muscular, hence active and energetic. All persons are classified as a mixture of these fundamental "types," graded as to predominance on a scale of 1 to 7.

*Unconscious*: 1. In general, any behavioral process of which the subject is not directly aware. In addition, *unconscious* has many meanings as variously used in the literature, ranging from stuporous to vaguely mystic connotations of atavistic communality (C. Jung, N. Miller). 2. In psychoanalytic topography, that portion of the *psyche* that comprises the Id instincts, plus those functions of the Ego (adaptive) and Superego (self-directive) that are in contact with the Id, and which are not available to direct awareness (*consciousness*) or immediate recall and introspection (*pre-conscious*) (Chapter 8).

*Undoing*: A defensive reversal of an anxiety-ridden act (Chapter 9).

*Ur-Defenses (-Delusions, -Illusions)*: Irrational but indestructible faiths in one's own (1) physical powers, (2) supposed friends, and (3) magical concepts and practices (Chapters 5 and 8).

*Voyeurism*: Excessive pleasure in seeing the opposite sex partially or wholly nude.

*Working-Through*: 1. In general, an active reexploration of a problem situation until satisfactory solutions or adaptations are found and firmly established. 2. In psychoanalysis, the tracing of a symbolism to its "deepest" unconscious sources.

*Zeigarnik Phenomenon*: The drive to complete an unfinished task (B. Zeigarnik, 1927).

# REFERENCES

Adler, A. *The practice and theory of individual psychology.* New York: Harcourt, 1924.

Alexander, F. *Fundamentals of psychoanalysis.* New York: Norton, 1948.

Alonso, A. & Ruton J.C. Object relation theory. *American Journal of Psychiatry* 1984, 141:1375-79.

American Psychiatric Association Commission on Psychiatric Therapies. *The psychiatric therapies.* Washington, D.C., 1984.

Armand, A.D. *Follow-up studies in psychotherapy.* New York: Transactional Mental Health Newsletter, 22:1-4, 1980.

Barrett, W. *What is Existentialism?* New York: Grove, 1964.

Bromberg, W. *From shaman to psychotherapist.* Chicago: Henry Regnery, 1975.

Carroll, B.J. Problems with diagnostic criteria. *Journal of Clinical Psychiatry,* 1984, 45:14-18.

Denber, H.C.B. *Textbook of clinical psychopharmacology, Serial handbook of modern psychiatry* (Vol. 3). New York: Stratton Intercontinental, 1979, pp. 135-164.

Ehrenwald, J. *From medicine man to Freud.* New York: Dell, 1956.

Eherenwald, J. *The history of psychotherapy.* New York: Jason Aronson, 1976.

Ellenberger, H. *The discovery of the unconscious: The history and evolution of dynamic psychiatry.* New York: Basic Books, 1970

Freud, S. *Outline of psychoanalysis.* New York: Norton, 1963.

Glass, G. *The benefits of psychotherapy.* Baltimore: Johns Hopkins Press, 1980.

Gold, M.S., & Verebey K. Pharmacology of cocaine. *Psychiatriac Annual,* 1984, *14*:114-118.

Hardin, G. *Nature and man's fate.* New York: Mentor, 1959.

Kiev, A. *Magic, faith and healing.* New York: Free Press, 1964.

Kohut, H. *The resotration of the self.* New York: International Universities Press, 1977.

London, P. *Behavior control.* New York: Harper & Row, 1970.

Marmor, J. *Modern psychoanalysis.* New York: Basic Books, 1968.

Masserman, J.H. *Neurosis and alcohol.* Motion picture film, 16 mm., subtitled. University Park, PA: Psychological Cinema Register, 1943.

Masserman, J.H. *Principles of dynamic psychiatry.* Philadelphia: Saunders, 1946.

Masserman, J.H. Faith and delusions in psychotherapy: The Ur-delusions of man. *American Journal of Psychiatry,* 1953, *110*:324-333.

Masserman, J.H. *Practice of dynamic psychiatry.* Philadelphia: Saunders, 1955.

Masserman, J.H. Say Id isn't so—with music. In J.H. Masserman (Ed.). *Science and Psychoanalysis,* Vol. 1, New York: Grune & Stratton, 1958a, pp. 76-187.

Masserman, J.H. Science, psychiatry and religion. In J.H. Masserman & J. Moreno. *Progress in Psychotherapy.* New York: Grune & Stratton, 1958b, pp. 97-99.

Masserman, J.H. *Behavior and neurosis* (3rd ed.). New York: Hafner, 1964.

Masserman, J.H. (Ed.). *Handbook for psychiatric therapies.* New York: Grune & Stratton, 1966.

Masserman, J.H. *The biodynamic roots of human behavior.* Springfield, IL: Charles C. Thomas, 1968.

Masserman, J.H. *A psychiatric odyssey.* New York: Science House, 1971.

Masserman, J.H. *Psychiatric syndromes and modes of therapy.* New York: Stratton Intercontinental, 1974.

Masserman, J.H. (Ed.). *The range of normal in human behavior.* New York: Grune & Stratton, 1976.

Masserman, J.H. Threescore and thirteen psychiatric therapies: An integration. In J.H. Masserman (Ed.), *Current Psychiatric Therapies* (Vol. 18). New York: Grune & Stratton, 1978.

Masserman, J.H. Presidential Address to the American Psychiatric Association. *American Journal of Psychiatry*, 1979, *137*:1013-1019.

*Masserman, J.H. The comparative scientific states of psychiatry. In J.H. Masserman (Ed.), Current Psychiatric Therapies* (Vol. 20). New York: Grune & Stratton, 1981, pp. 3–15.

Masserman, J.H. Biodynamics. In H.I. Kaplan, A.M. Freedman, & B.J. Sadock (Eds.). *Comprehensive textbook of psychiatry*, (3rd ed.) Baltimore: Williams & Wilkins, 1982a, pp. 782–789.

Masserman, J.H. The common dynamics of therapy and their presumed results. In J.H. Masserman, (Ed.), *Current psychiatric therapies* (Vol. 21). New York: Grune & Stratton, 1982b, pp. 20–33.

Masserman, J.H., et al. 18 Motion picture films (16mm, subtitled or sound) on the life development, neurophysiology, social interactions, reactions to alcohol and other drugs, neurotigenesis, and modes of therapy in various animal species. University Park, PA: Psychological Cinema Register, 1940.

Masserman, J.H., & Schwab, J.J. (eds.). *The psychiatric examination.* New York: Intercontinental Medical Books, 1974.

Meyer, A. *Collected works of Adolf Meyer* (4 vols.). E.E. Winters, (Ed.). Baltimore: Johns Hopkins Press, 1950–52.

Miller, J.G. *Living systems.* New York: McGraw-Hill, 1978.

National Institute of Mental Health. Mental state of the Union. *Newsweek,* October 15, 1984, p. 113.

Parloff, M.B., Research in therapists' variables. In S.L. Garfield & A.E. Bergin (Eds.). *Handbook of psychotherapy.* New York: Wiley 1979.

Salzman, L., & Masserman, J.H. (Eds.). *Modern concepts of psychoanalysis.* New York: Philosophical Library, 1968.

Sartorius, N. Diagnosis and classification. *Mental Health & Society*, 1978, *5*:79-85.

Schmitt W. *The origin and growth of religion.* New York: Humanities Press, 1935.

Schwab J.J. Psychiatric manifestations of infectious diseases. In R.C.W. Hall (Ed.). *Psychiatric presentation of medical illness.* New York: Wiley, 1980.

Waterman, P.F. *The story of superstition.* New York: Knopf, 1929.

Wiener, J.M. *Psychopharmocology in childhood and adolescence.* New York: Jason Aronson, 1978.

Wolberg, L.R. *Techniques of psychotherapy.* (2 Vols., 3rd. ed.) New York: Grune & Stratton, 1967, 1978.

Yalom, I. *The theory and practice of group psychotherapy.* New York: Basic Books, 1975.

# INDEX OF NAMES

Ackerman, N., 112
Adler, A., 90, 241
Agras, W.S., 108
Ahriman, 92
Alexander, F., 11, 89, 93, 95, 241
Alger, I., 112
Alonso, A., 241
Anaximander, 21
Angelicus, Fra, 32
Apollo, 22
Aristotle, 22
Armand, A.D., 241
Ayllon, T., 106
Azrin, N.H., 106

Bahrdedarma, Buddha, 103
Barber, T.X., 96, 122
Barrett, W., 241
Bateson, G., 92
Beers, C., 31
Bellak, A., 101

Berne, E., 114
Bierer, J., 31
Binswanger, L., 98
Birk, C.L., 122
Boccacio, 96
Brahma, 93
Brill, H., 77
Brocque, L., 134
Bromberg, W., 241
Bruno, G., 27
Buber, M., 98
Burton, R., 98

Camus, A., 22, 98
Carrington, P., 102
Carrol, R.S., 30
Carroll, B.J., 55, 241
Casriel, T., 113
Cassirer, E., 27
Chase, M., 111
Chi, W., 101

Chiarugi, V., 30
Chrzanowsky, G., 91
Colby, K., 97
Comte, A., 47
Cone, E., 96
Corson, S.A., 97, 103
Cotton, H., 30
Crowley, R., 91
Cummings, N., 62

Denber, H.C.B., 241
Descartes, R., 27
Dewey, J., 77
Diderich, C., 114
Dix, D., 30
Draper, G., 238
Dubois, W., 99
Duns Scotus, J., 27
Dwyer, T., 102

Eddy, M.B., 28, 116
Ehrenwald, J., 117, 241
Eisenbud, J., 98
Ellenberger, J., 32, 242
Ellis, A., 100
Enelow, G., 100
Engedu, 93
Erhard, W., 112
Esquirrol, J.E., 29

Falret, I.P., 47
Fay, A., 99
Feldenkreis, M., 100
Fenwick, S., 118
Ferenczi, S., 92
Ferguson, J.M., 107
Freud, S., 31, 77, 88, 97, 98, 242
Fromm, E., 86

Galen, 238
Gall, F.J., 30
Gardner, R.A., 97
Garma, A., 91
Gaston, E.T., 113
Gesell, A., 93
Gill, M., 132
Glass, A., 113
Glass, G., 242
Glass, L.L., 118
Glueck, B., 96
Gold, M.S., 242
Goldenson, R.M., 97
Goulden, R.L., 101
Gralnick, A., 112
Graves, R., 133
Greatrakes, V., 28

Hall, G., 77
Halleck, S., 113
Hardin, G., 242
Harlow, H., 92
Harper, R., 100
Hart, J., 97
Hatcher, C., 112
Hegel, G.W., 22, 27
Heisenberg, W., 27
Heraclitus, 22
Hippocrates, 22
Hirai, T., 102
Hoch, P., 235
Horney, K., 86, 89
Hubbard, L.R., 97
Hudolin, V., 31

Ibn' Sennah, 26

Jackson, D., 98
Jacobson, E., 96, 101

Jacquet, L., 134
James, W., 77
Joan of Arc, 54
Jung, C., 77, 91, 98

Kafka, F., 27
Kahlbaum, K., 47
Kant, I., 27
Karasu, B., 62
Kardiner, A., 86
Kelman, H., 113
Khayyam, O., 98
Kierkegaard, S., 27, 98
Kiev, A., 242
Klein, M., 91
Knobloch, J., 113
Kohler, W., 113
Kohut, H., 94, 242
Kors, P., 100
Kostrubala, T., 112
Kuhn, C.C., 142

Lacan, J., 91
Lanbaurn, J., 132
Langsley, D., 111
Laqueur, H.P., 112
Leary, T., 102
Lesse, S., 62
Lester, D., 102
Levy, D., 81
Lewis, A., 31
Liddell, H., 104
Linn, L., 99
Linne, C. von, 47
Loki, 92
Lombroso, C., 30
Lomont, R., 107
London, P., 62, 242
Lorand, S., 81

Low, A., 96, 114
Lowen, A., 96

Mahler, M., 89
Malinowsky, B., 92
Malleck, S., 62
Maltz, M., 100
Marcus, E., 112
Marcus, I., 96
Marmor, J., 62, 100, 242
Maxmen, J., 97
Mazda, A., 93
Mead, M., 92, 93
Medvedev, Z., 116
Meldmann, M.J., 95
Menninger, R., 54
Mesmer, A., 28, 32, 73
Meyer, A., 11, 30, 47, 243
Michelangelo, 19
Miller, J.G., 243
Miller, N.E., 104
Mitchell, W., 101
Morita, 99
Moses, ben Maimon, 26

Naumberg, M., 96, 110
Nemiah, J., 62
Nietzche, F.W., 27

Ogburn, W.F., 47
Osiris, M., 93
Osler, W., 134

Parloff, M.B., 243
Paul, I.H., 97
Pavlov, I., 104
Perls, F., 112
Peters, J., 93

Pichot, P., 31
Pierce, C., 77
Pinel, P., 29
Pittenger, R.E., 96
Plato, 22
Pliny the Elder, 22
Price, R., 111
Pythagoras, 21

Ra, 93
Rado, S., 31, 235
Rainer, J., 112
Rajneesh, Bhagwan Shree, 111
Rank, O., 91, 100
Rawcliffe, D., 98
Ray, Isaac, 30
Reich, W., 92, 96, 102
Rheder, H., 102
Ricoh, J., 31
Rogers, C., 97
Rolf, I., 101
Rosenheim, E., 98
Rush, B., 33, 106
Ruton, J.C., 241

Salzman, L., 243
Santayana, G., 27
Sartorius, N., 243
Sartre, J.P., 27, 98
Saslow, G., 97
Satan, 92
Schmidt, W., 31, 243
Schultz, J.H., 95
Schwab, J.J., 13, 142, 243
Sechenov, I., 104
Selma, A., 98
Seth, 92
Shakespeare, W., 96
Shorr, J., 100
Silva, J., 98
Simon, J., 118

Skinner, B.F., 104
Sophocles, 23
Speck, R.V., 112
Sperry, R., 55
Spiegel, J., 54
Spinoza, B., 27
St. Augustine, 26
Sullivan, H.S., 86, 91

Theophrastus, 22
Thoreau, H., 27
Treffert, D.V., 101
Tschazo, O., 110
Tuke, W., 30
Tyndell, M., 99

Vahia, N., 103
Vaillant, G., 54
Verebez, K., 242
Viner, H., 30
Voegtlin, M., 106

Walter, B., 86
Waterman, P., 62, 243
Wayne, G., 111
Weier, J., 27
Weimer, W.B., 107
Weinroth, J., 99
Weir-Mitchell, S., 33
Wittson, C., 102
Wolberg, L.R., 101, 121, 244
Wolpe, J., 108

Yalom, I., 244
Yaweh, 93
Yogi, Maharishi Mahesh, 102
Yogi, Rami, 103

Zegans, L.S., 101

# INDEX OF SUBJECTS

Adolescence, 82, 149
Affect, 85, 205
Aggressivity, 79
Aging, 156, 186
Akathisia, 205
Alcoholism, 172
Alexander technique, 95
Alzheimer's disease, 205
Ambivalence, 205
Amentia, 205
American Psychiatric Association, 31, 193, 204
Amnesia, 205
Amytal narcosis, 121
Anorexia nervosa, 189, 206
Antidepressants, 127
Anxiety, 50, 137, 160, 206
Anxiolytics, 124
Aphasia, 206
Assertiveness training, 107
Attention antenna, 95
Aura, 207

Autism, 147
Autogenic training, 95
Auto-hypnosis, 96
Automation, 207
Autosuggestion, 96
Aversion techniques, 106

Biodynamics, 56ff., 207
Biofeedback, 96
Birth trauma, 78

Catharsis, 208
Celestial bed, 159
Childhood, 66, 148, 193
Christian Science Church, 28, 116
Climacterium, 154
Clinical examination, 34ff.
Commission on Therapies, 58
Community services, 110
Compulsions, 69

Computer feedback, 97
Conations, 65
Confidentiality, 64
Congenital abnormalities, 146
Conscience, 86
Contingency contracts, 107
Conversion reactions, 85
Cornelian Corner, 92
Countertransference, 210
Criminality, 168, 210
Cultural influences, 86, 93

Déjà vu, 211
Delirium, 211
Denial, 84, 138
Depression, 139, 182, 212
Depressive syndromes, 51
Desensitization, 105
Deterrence, 106
Diagnosis, 17, 45
Dialysis, 122
Dianetics, 97
Directiveness, 65
Disorders
   affective, 200
   factitious, 202
   neurotic, 199
   organic, 201
   personality, 203
   somatiform, 204
Displacement, 84
Do In, 97
Down's Syndrome, 213
Dramatics, 23
Dreams, 66
DSM III, 48, 193
Dukhobors, 54
Duplicity, 71
Dying, 159

Ego, 83, 94
Ego defenses, 84

Ego-ideal, 87
Eidetic imagery, 214
Endocrines, 136
Epilepsy, 53, 135, 215
Ergasias, 30
Eroticism, 79, 149
Exercises, 101

Fantasy formation, 66, 85
Finger-painting, 96
Flooding, 107
Formulation, psychiatric, 45
Fugue, 217

Ganser Syndrome, 217
General paresis, 218
Genetics, 147
Genius, 147
Grief, 138
Guilt, 70

Habits, 69
Hate, 70
Health, 16
Hebrews, 26
Heredity, 39
Holy Rollers, 54
Hypnosis, 73ff
Hypomania, 182
Hysteria, 219

Id, 83
Identity, 151
Infancy, 145
Insanity, 220
Insight, 43, 88, 220
Institutionalization, 158
Integrations, 15ff.

Intellect, 42
Intelligence, 220
Introjects, 91, 93
Irrelevancy, 38
Irresistible impulses, 69

Jargon, 70

Korsakoff Psychosis, 221
Krishna Consciousness, 103

*La belle indifference*, 189
Lao Tze, 32
Latent period, 81
Libido, 78
Lithium, 127
Living Love, 98
Love, 70, 222

Malingering, 222
*Malleus Maleficarum*, 27, 32
M'Naughten rule, 223
Masochism, 222
Mental status, 42
Metapsychiatry, 98
Mind control, 98
Mores, 93
Motivations, 64
Music, 23

Narcissism, 78
Narcolepsy, 224
Neuroses, 51, 169, 225
Nirvana fantasy, 225

Obsessive-compulsive reactions,
   85

Occam's Razor, 19
Oedipus complex, 23, 80, 209
Operant conditioning, 102
Organic impairments, 53
Orgone boxes, 92
Orthopsychiatry, 226

Pain, 185
Panic, 166
Paranoid states, 52
Persona, 228
Personalities, borderline, 51, 89
Personality, 16, 83, 228
Persuasion, 99
Pharmacotoxic states, 52
Phobias, 85
Phobic-obsessive-compulsive
   syndromes, 50
Physical examination, 44
Play techniques, 97
Postoedipal development, 81
Primal scene, 80
Primal scream, 97
Prognosis, 17
Projection, 85
Promiscuity, 150
Psyche, 15, 18
Psychoanalysis, 77ff.
   concepts, 78
   Ego defenses, 84
   personality structure, 83
   schools, 89
   techniques, 88
Psychobiology, 230
Psychoimagination, 100
Psychological tests, 44
Psychopharmacology, 124ff.
Psychophysiologic disturbances,
   51
Psychoses, 53, 230
Psychosomatics, 85
Puberty, 82, 148

Rapport, 59
Reaction formation, 84
Reality principle, 233
Recycling, 61, 71
Regression, 85, 138, 149
Rehabilitation, 141
REM sleep, 233
Reorientation, 153
Repression, 84
Resistances, 67, 233
Resocialization, 61, 141
Responsibility, 64
Rest cures, 101
Rolfing, 101
Ruminations, 66

Sanatoria, 22
Scatology, 80
Schizophrenia, 176, 179, 234
Scientology, 97
Self-analysis, 94
Semantics, 69
Sensorium, 43
Sexuality, 66
Sociopathic personality, 168, 235
Sublimation, 84
Substitution, 84
Superego, 86
Suppression, 84

T'ai Chi, 101
Telepsychiatry, 102
Temple of Health, 159
Therapies, 17
  adolescence, 149
  aging, 159
  antinarcotic, 122
  Arica, 110
  art, 110
  behavior, 104ff.

  child, 96, 148
  climacterium, 154
  clothing, 97
  costs, 68
  costume, 96
  counting, 97
  crisis, 111
  dance, 111
  dyadic, 95ff.
  dynamic, 59
  electrocerebral, 123
  electrosleep, 124
  electrostimulation, 124
  Erhard seminar training, 112
  Esalin, 111
  exercise, 112
  existential, 98
  experimental, 56
  faith healings, 117
  family, 112, 186
  genetic counseling, 112
  geriatric, 112
  gestalt, 112
  Greek, 22
  group, 71, 109ff.
  infancy, 145
  integrated, 113
  interactional, 98
  introduction, 63ff.
  marathon, 113
  marital, 151, 164
  mentor, 98
  metapsychologic, 116ff.
  middle years, 153
  milieu, 111
  military, 113
  Morita, 99, 107
  music, 113
  mystic, 117
  narcotherapy, 124
  nonagenic, 99
  occupational, 99

paradoxical, 99
penal, 113
pet, 97
physical, 133ff.
poetry, 99
posture, 100
preview, 56ff.
psychoanalytic, 88
puberty, 148
puppet, 100
rational-emotive, 100
redecision, 101
religious healings, 117
review, 143
results, 192
self-help groups, 114
sexual, 151
social skill, 101
somatic, 119ff., 139
supportive, 101
Syanon, 114
tantric, 99
termination, 72
transactional, 114
transcendental meditation, 102

transference, 237
various ages, 143ff.
vectors, 191
vegetotherapy, 102
work, 116
Z, 116
zootherapy, 103
Types, character, 237

Undoing, 84
Ur concepts, 17, 21, 50, 63, 143,
190, 239

World Association for Social Psychiatry, 31

Yoga, 98, 103

Zazen, 102
Zeigarnik phenomenon, 239
Zen, 103